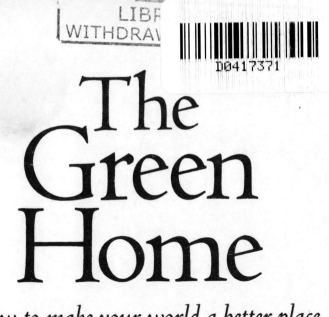

The Green Home

How to make your world a better place

KAREN CHRISTENSEN

PIATKUS

First published as *Home Ecology* in 1989 by
Arlington Books (Publishers) Ltd, London

This edition first published in 1995 by
Judy Piatkus (Publishers) Ltd of
5 Windmill Street, London W1P 1HF

**The moral rights of the author
have been asserted**

*A catalogue record of this book is
available from the British Library*

ISBN 0–7499 1460–2

Edited by Carol Franklin
Designed by Sue Ryall
Illustrations by Judy Strafford and Zena Flax

Typeset by Computerset, Harmondsworth, Middlesex
Printed and bound in Great Britain by
Mackays of Chatham PLC

CONTENTS

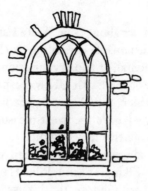

Acknowledgements

In 1988 I knew far more about 'The Waste Land' than I did about the ozone layer or sustainable agriculture, so I must acknowledge the many environmentalists and organizations who educated and guided me. Friends of the Earth UK was especially helpful. The enthusiasm with which the Women's Environmental Network adopted *Home Ecology* gave me great pleasure and I appreciate their help in preparing this new edition.

Many people encouraged me with their enthusiasm for *The Green Home*. John Elkington and Julia Hailes deserve special mention for their willingness to discuss the issue of consumerism. Other people – notably Alan Durning of the Worldwatch Institute, Satish Kumar of *Resurgence* and Sandy Irvine of the *Ecologist* – reinforced my conviction that *The Green Home* should concentrate on how we live, not what we buy. There are few joys greater than to hear that a book has changed someone's life, and I am deeply grateful to readers who have written to share their stories with me. Amongst them, Caroline Bennett and Sue Ross stand out for their enthusiasm and commitment.

The research required to update a book on ever-changing issues would not have been possible without the patient work and astute observations of freelance editor Pamela Dix. I am grateful to librarian Chris Dagg of Woking for updating the bibliography and to Jean Macqueen for the fine index. Tessa Strickland of Barefoot Books has been a firm supporter and friend and she has brought out my first children's book, *Rachel's Roses*, to coincide with publication of *The Green Home* – for me, an experience like having twins!

A book is a team effort, demanding more work from more people than most readers would ever guess. At Piatkus Books I want to thank Judy Piatkus, Gill Cormode, Nina Webley, Jana Sommerlad, and Carol Franklin for all that they have done to make *The Green Home* what it is.

My husband David has been known to turn green at the mention of *The Green Home*, but his encouragement and patience have never wavered. He, Tom and Rachel have my gratitude and love.

FOREWORD

by Jonathon Porritt

When Karen Christensen's *Home Ecology* first came out in 1989, this country was almost at the height of its 'green consumer frenzy'. People had leapt from doing all but nothing to thinking they could do everything overnight. The most improbable organizations and publications were suddenly offering 'green tips' of every description, and the most questionable companies were trumpeting their slimline green credentials as if they were going out of fashion.

Thankfully, they did go out of fashion! The frenzy subsided, the dishonest claims and madly-hyped advertising slogans became more of a liability than a smart marketing strategy and, once again, commentators were able to get a proper perspective on the role of green consumerism as just one aspect of a much wider and more complex social movement.

But people did *not* lose interest. The environment may have become 'yesterday's issue' to much of the media, but for huge numbers of people it remains an enormously important area of concern. Regular polls and sampling by organizations like MORI and Mintel have confirmed this phenomenon throughout the first half of the 1990s.

What is true is that a lot of people became confused and uncertain about the value of what they were doing as individuals. At the same time they were cynical about the motives of government ministers and business leaders who were constantly exhorting the public to get out there and save the earth. Green consumerism, as a stand-alone politically detached game plan for setting the world to rights, became discredited. And properly so.

Neither *Home Ecology* nor *The Green Home* (its comprehensive and timely rewrite for the 1990s) falls into that trap. Individual lifestyle choices, arising out of an acceptance of personal responsibility for those parts of our lives that we *can* control, are set in a much broader social, political and philosophical context. As Karen Christensen says, 'This is not a green consumer guide. It's about better living, not better buying.' And better living means thinking of ourselves primarily as *citizens* (be it of our local community or of planet earth itself) and only after that as consumers.

Even as we reduce our energy consumption, buy more organic produce, and eliminate the last of those chemicals we might once have used in the garden, we must not ignore the political side: the letter-writing, the joining of others in local or national campaigns, the encouraging of best practice wherever we find it, etc.

Both aspects of 'being green' – the practical and the political – are essential. Each depends on the other. And that's very much where *The Green Home* is coming from. One of the things that I like best about *The Green Home* is that (unlike many books) it won't make concerned and committed people feel inadequate or paralysed by guilt! Though it reminds me of endless shortcomings in my own lifestyle (busy green activists are often far from the paragons of environmental virtue that they might aspire to be – and no one aspires more than I do!), it encourages rather than turns me off.

As the author says, there's no point being 'grim and miserable' if you are seeking a greener way of life and a greener home. At its simplest (but most easily overlooked) level, environmentalism is all about celebrating the gift of life – life writ large, that is, not just the human end of it. Better by far to be celebrating that gift wreathed in smiles than permanently garbed in sackcloth and ashes. To celebrate, for instance, the joy of good fresh food rather than becoming obsessed by what we should or shouldn't be eating.

Karen Christensen declares that her secret to happiness is 'not getting more but wanting less'. I suspect that she and I are still working away at this secret. *The Green Home* is about work in progress, not about some revealed truth from a distant green guru – and it is all the more useful and enjoyable for it.

Jonathon Porritt

INTRODUCTION

When I was thirteen my father started what he called 'ecology runs'. He would muster as many kids as possible and drive into the foothills above California's Santa Clara Valley to gather rubbish which had been thrown along the roadside. Cans went to the recycling centre, bottles went to the grocery store and the rest was bagged for collection. Dad glowed with accomplishment.

I hated the word *ecology* and never once went on an ecology run. Dad's quiet statement of civic responsibility was too tame for me, and trash was messy. I was unable to see a connection between the state of the roads and the state of my world. Only after my son was born in London in 1985 did it dawn on me that my concern about his well-being and future was connected with the environmental issues I read about in the paper each morning.

Within a year, I had a contract for *Home Ecology*, quit my publishing job and became a freelance environmental writer and occasional activist. I later dived into the debate over green consumerism, and began researching a new book on the search for community. I continued to be deeply interested in ideas about lifestyle change, while my own life has changed dramatically. I've struggled to put principles into practice, first as a single mother with two preschool children and more recently juggling a demanding job, new home and new husband.

I was glad to see green issues enter the mainstream. Nowadays, when I say I'm an environmental writer, people complain about the recycling facilities in their neighbourhoods and my friends no longer see me as a crank. (E. F. Schumacher, the author of *Small Is Beautiful*, was happy to be called a crank. He explained that cranks are small, efficient tools that make revolutions.)

But I was disappointed to see the proliferation of silly suggestions for green living such as 'write small so you use less paper', or 'squeeze lemon juice into your washing machine to whiten clothes'. *The Green Home* is more realistic. It is full of information to guide you to making practical choices about everyday things – washing the dishes, feeding the dog, or choosing a holiday destination.

As you read, mark the ideas you want to try. Make the book your own. Although I would be happy if you read *The Green Home* from cover to cover, I would prefer you to have it sitting within easy reach, beside your favourite cookbooks.

Sources of further information – books, journals, and green organizations – are listed at the end of the book. In this edition I have included only organizations which have been around for a couple of years. Larger organizations can put you in touch with more specialist groups. I have added suggestions for greening the office to several chapters because more and more of us work, part time or full time, in our homes.

I'd love to hear from readers with further ideas and suggestions for *The Green Home*. Write c/o Piatkus Books, 5 Windmill Street, London W1P 1HF or via e-mail at: christensen@external umass.edu.

1

TIME

When I began work on *The Green Home*, I told a close friend that I was researching things each of us could do to solve environment problems. I expected her to be enthusiastic and was surprised that she was defensive: 'I care, of course,' she said, 'but I don't have time to do anything extra. I wish I did.' Her life was so full and sometimes so difficult, with two children and a job to juggle, that she thought I was going to make her feel guilty about not doing enough.

Surveys show that women, and mothers in particular, are the group most concerned about the environment. But they are the people who have least time to spare. One survey of working mothers found that they talked about sleep as a starving person talks about food. When I suggest switching to cloth nappies or making soup with kitchen leftovers, their first reaction is often, 'I don't have time for things like that!'

I, too, have children, husband and job, as well as aspirations to find a little time for myself, and I decided to start *The Green Home* with a chapter about time because our waking hours are what we start with, in any new venture, on any new path. Before looking at particular environmental issues, we need to think about how we can find the time and energy to make changes in the way we live. After all, the way we spend our time is a reflection of our values.

Our attitude towards time influences how we go about caring for our homes. Wandering round the house early in the morning when everyone else is asleep – opening curtains to the day, tidying newspapers, bringing in the milk, making a pot of tea – can be a hurried chore or a ritual you love, a way to reconnect with the details and rhythms of your home and place.

Creating a home and way of life which, while not perfect, is full of magic and charm for you, as well as for other people, is one of the most important expenditures of time you can make. The steps you take in creating a green home should be the result of care, not fear, a matter of nurturing things you love and admire, not barricading yourself and your family from things you dislike or disapprove of.

Only you can decide about your own days and years, and taking time to consider how you want to spend the time of your life is the first step in creating your green home. You may also worry that a green home is going to cost too much, so the next chapter deals with the second half of the Time + Money equation. But first let's look at the way time – or our perception of it – makes us tick.

THE TIME OF YOUR LIFE

Although we often say that time is money, if every moment spent relaxing, playing with your children or contemplating the ocean waves were a penny lost, every human activity could be quantified in terms of its monetary value. How much is your baby's smile worth, or a game of chess or helping a ten year old with her maths homework? How about a day spent decorating the house for Christmas or an afternoon in bed with your beloved?

Money can sometimes buy time – by making it possible, for example, to hire someone to do a task you dislike or aren't good at – but the idea that time is money is misleading. People end up trapped by the need to finance a luxurious lifestyle and may in fact have far less free time than those who live more simply. E. F. Schumacher, the former Coal Board economist who became internationally renowned as the author of *Small is Beautiful – Economics as if people mattered*, summed this up with what he called the first law of economics, 'The amount of real leisure a society enjoys tends to be in inverse proportion to the amount of labour-saving machinery it employs' and, presumably, to the amount of money it has. In the same way, the more money a society has, the less real leisure time people enjoy.

Contrary to the notion that we have more free time than our ancestors, a notion fostered by a culture which needs our continual contribution as employees and as consumers, people in some primitive agricultural or hunter–gatherer societies actually enjoyed more leisure than we do. As a rule, they spent between 15 and 20 hours a week providing for themselves and their children, leaving the remainder of their time for socializing and relaxing. (This is not the case for many third world women today, however; the chores of obtaining scarce water and firewood take up an increasingly large proportion of their day.)

Many people who live directly off the earth find considerable amounts of time to engage in activities that are not economic: enjoying religious rituals, fiestas and pow-wows, arranging marriages, renewing friendships. In Victorian novels, even working people seemed to find time for festivities at county fairs and on market days. Our free time is less leisurely and more expensive than that of our grandparents. It is also less simple to decide how to spend our leisure time because our lives are complicated by multiple roles, and by our beepers, computerized diaries and cellular phones. A Sunday afternoon ramble and pub lunch have to be squeezed between catching up with the weekly washing and finishing off a report for Monday's staff meeting. To be important in today's world, we have to be busy.

TIME PRESSURES

While small children and double shifts are obvious causes of exhaustion, the feeling that you don't have time for new activities or to make changes in your life may be the result of stress, rather than a realistic assessment of your life. Underneath superficial energy is often a weariness we can't seem to shake off. Count the people you know who are really healthy and vibrant, full of energy and enthusiasm. Isn't it surprising that more people don't fit that description, considering our affluence and our knowledge about good eating habits and exercise? But the weariness that comes from a high pressured or much hated job – requiring much wind-down time – has little to do with physical fatigue. Fatigue and depression are also common symptoms of environmental stresses, which range from poor diet or working in a modern 'sick' office block, to a sensitivity to household chemicals. In one way or another, the way we live is to blame.

Look, too, at some of the bigger issues in your life. Why do you work and live where you do? How do you travel to work? What about your health – how do you feel most of the time? How happy are you? All these things are interrelated, and need to be considered as you take on the ideas and suggestions in *The Green Home*.

CONSUMERS OF CONVENIENCE

Our need to do things faster has led to a vast increase in convenience products, from frozen meals and fast-drying paint to permanent-press clothes. We have been sold the idea of convenience, because a sense of urgency and helplessness about everyday chores is one way of increasing consumer demand. The cost of this convenience is a loss of quality, along with a number of environmental price tags. Journalist Erik Larson quipped, 'As far as food engineers are concerned, the microwave oven is one lousy cooking device but consumers are very forgiving when it comes to microwave foods. They readily swap quality for speed.'

As we consider the quality of life we want, however, our priorities may change. The time-saving nature of convenience products is often illusory. Natural rice needs to cook for longer than the instant variety but its preparation requires no more of your time. Cooking and sharing a meal, and doing the dishes

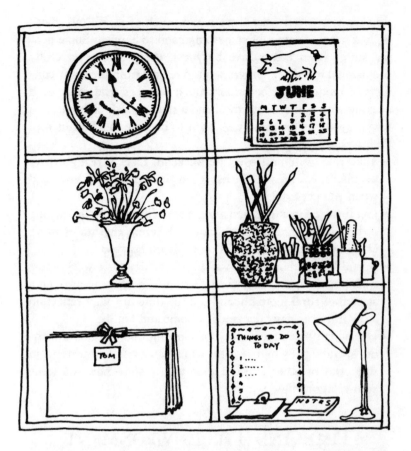

afterwards takes more time than sticking individual frozen pizzas into the microwave, but eating together plays a vital role in any human group, and shared preparation is both creative and pleasurable. Think of the extent to which friendships are built up by years of shared experiences. Taking a child to a museum or building a dolls' house together is likely to mean far more in later years than any number of purchased toys.

TIME VALUES

Beyond this, we all have patterns of time use that may not reflect what we really want and value in our lives. We talk about 'quality time', which means that there is not much of it. We talk about 'killing time', waiting for something good to happen. Some people suffer from compulsive busyness, every minute carefully preplanned in a diary. Others want to retreat from the many conflicts of modern life, becoming couch potatoes who retire each evening with a microwave meal and a stack of videos. Here are a few suggestions for those who want to become more attuned to the passage of time:

▶ Take your watch off over the weekend. Does it really matter whether it is 2:36 or 2:39? Eat when you feel hungry; go to bed when you get tired.

▶ Get involved in a time-consuming craft like pottery or knitting or bookbinding, and get to know a different rhythm of work, creating something that will probably outlast you.

▶ Spend half an hour or so walking every day for a week – just walking, not going anywhere. Get to know your area or a stretch of rural footpath, and use the time for quiet reflection away from the daily demands of home and family.

▶ Do something extraordinary for someone you care about without spending any money. This will mean a gift of your time, in some way or other, and is a good way to show how you value your relationships.

TIME AND THE ENVIRONMENT

As more and more of us use increasingly powerful computers, psychologists and sociologists, as well as environmentalists, are expressing concern about the effect this new perception of time will have on our relationships with each other and with the environment. They say that our obsession with speed has gone too far and that the desire, especially of the Western world, to produce and consume at a frantic pace has led to social inequalities as well as to the depletion of natural resources and the pollution we see around us. Nature's own production and recycling rhythms cannot keep up with modern industrial society. The demands of economic efficiency and ever-increasing speed mean that planetary ecosystems[1] are no longer capable of renewing resources as fast as they are being depleted, or recycling waste as fast as we discard it.

We read less, watch television more, and want our news and information in smaller bites, to grab on the run. Environmentalists complain that people won't understand the complex choices of our modern society without taking more time to listen and learn. But this is becoming a world of soundbites in which our choices, our decisions and our behaviour are too often determined by quick takes rather than serious consideration.

US activist Jeremy Rifkin points out that computers are making changes in the social, physiological and political dimensions of the way we perceive time. Computers measure time in nanoseconds, billionths of a second, which we can conceive of theoretically but which we cannot experience. 'Never before,' says Rifkin, 'has time been organized at a speed beyond the realm of consciousness.'

These changes have happened, in part, because of the Western idea of time as linear, with a separate past, present and future, with the present being the most important. Other cultures – including the Hindu, Chinese and many Native American cultures – have a circular view of time. Because they believe that what they do in the present affects the lives of others, and their own lives in the future, they have been more likely to live lightly in the present.

TECHNOLOGY

While many environmentalists extol the virtues of technological innovation – telecommuting, for example, and e-mail, and more efficient electrical appliances – others are uneasy about the mesmerizing effect of new technologies. Building computers uses

---

[1]An ecosystem is a community of plants, animals and microbes in one particular place, with its distinctive terrain, weather patterns etc. As it functions as an interconnected unit, if one part of the system is damaged or altered, the whole suffers.

rare natural resources, requires the use of many toxic chemicals (linked in California's Silicon Valley to congenital defects and miscarriage), consume an increasing amount of the world's energy and produce a great deal of waste. And they have not produced the paperless office, one of the benefits that was supposed to result from increased computerization. In fact, modern offices use more paper than ever before.

It is true that computers and computer networking are powerful tools for environmentalists. They facilitate fast, cheap communication as well as sophisticated monitoring of current problems and modelling of future environmental scenarios. But, social consequences aside, technological advance is devastating in terms of human consumption for the simple reason that every time computers get twice as fast and half the price, millions more people buy new machines. The same is true of fax machines, laser printers, telephones, ice-cream makers, CD players and the hundreds of other machines we use. The equipment we use is so complex, and changes so dramatically every few years, that it is not possible (or economically feasible) simply to adapt the old machine. And there is no end in sight, no satisfaction of need for the hacker, or the businesses who will always want to do things faster and cheaper.

The Amish, who use neither cars nor electricity, have long restricted the use of certain farm machinery because they value neighbourliness. If a machine replaces the need for the help of neighbours, they often choose not to use it because they value the human connection to be found in working together. Technology is always going to exclude people. Only a few people will have the latest and fastest, and technological advance takes no account of the fact that humans do not operate faster and faster. The idea of a quantum leap has no relationship with human lives, where change is slow, and where we value stability and familiarity.

If going faster means a loss of quality (artificial ripening of fruit), of human contacts (shopping by computer) and of human values (traditional village life, for example, and a responsible and responsive relationship with the place we live), we ought to think about slowing down, and we ought to slow down while we think.

CHRONOBIOLOGY

There is also a biological component to the way we live our days, hours and minutes. Plants, animals and human beings have inbuilt 'clocks'. Seasonal growth cycles, mating patterns and the way we wake up on New York time after a flight to London are examples of this.

Studies have found that the effects of a given drug can vary depending on the time of day it is administered. Long-distance truck drivers are three times as likely to have an accident at 5 am. The nuclear accident at Three Mile Island, Pennsylvania, occurred at 4 am, because of errors made by workers who had been rotating shifts around the clock every week for a month and a half.

Job satisfaction, general health and productivity were dramatically improved at a plant in Montana when a new schedule allowed workers to stay on the same shift for three weeks instead of one, and when the rotation went forward rather than backward; this makes a difference because most people's biological clock runs on a 25-hour rather than a 24-hour day. Shift work and jet lag can cause dramatic changes in mood and mental clarity, but trying to live by 'social time' can pose problems for people whose natural biorhythm has unsocial peaks and troughs.

Find your own prime time before you tackle the suggestions in the rest of *The Green Home*. If you aren't sure about your own biorhythms, consider the following.

▶ Are you more likely to feel chilled in the morning or the evening? Body temperature tends to peak along with alertness.

▶ Try doing a crossword puzzle at different times of the day. When is it easiest?

▶ Exercise for five minutes in the morning and again in the late afternoon or evening. Does one session leave you feeling exhausted and the other energized?

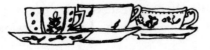

SIMPLIFY YOUR LIFE

While many authors have approached the idea of green living as a complicated enterprise requiring lots of extra equipment and a completely new programme, I think of it as a way of clarifying the things that really matter to me so I can simplify the rest and concentrate my effort (and my time and money) where it counts. Living more simply can bring dividends of leisure because you decide that you're just not going to bother doing some things any more!

Think about ways you might eliminate clutter from your home and about the worries or responsibilities that make for mental clutter. What can you get rid of, stop doing, do less often or get someone else – your partner, children or even hired help – to do? What can you do more simply? What about food, make-up, clothes, decorating, holidays?

The secret to happiness is not getting more but wanting less. Simplifying your life does not mean doing without things that really matter to you – the objects and activities that give you pleasure and satisfaction, and nourishment of soul and body – but doing without all the things you've been told you need which end up confusing the view, cluttering your cupboards and wasting your time.

There are more suggestions throughout *The Green Home*, but here is a basic list to help you begin to simplify your life.

► get rid of the clutter;
► rethink your buying habits;
► reduce your need for services;
► ask yourself whether the time you spend on upkeep (houseplants, pets, clothes, cars, appliances) is really worth the effort.

PLANNING

As I talked to people about *The Green Home* during the green boom of the early 1990s, I realized how many suggestions there were for 'ways to save the earth'. I felt overwhelmed by them. I did certain things and not others, and finally realized that I had to find a way to make decisions about what mattered most and what made most sense in my life.

A good idea is to start with things which are particularly easy or particularly important, and perhaps both (boycotting chloro-fluorocarbons (CFCs), for example). A few things cost a substantial amount of money (like building a conservatory). Some depend on the cooperation of the people you live with and should probably be left for later in the process of creating a green home.

Set priorities. Don't become overwhelmed by the prospect of filtering your water, changing cleaning products and spending more time in natural light, all in one week. Specialize. Decide what matters to you or bothers you most. Concentrate on the things you will enjoy, such as finding good second-hand furniture for your new flat or tuning your car engine for improved efficiency.

Many people find it helpful to start a household notebook, where you can keep track of ideas to try and questions which come to mind as you read. You can also note down healthy, easy vegetarian recipes and knitting patterns you cut from magazines, and plan your steps in creating a green home.

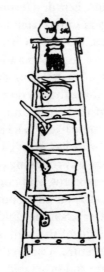

For instance, planning your meals is a great aid to ecological eating. Menus do not have to be complicated or too detailed. I find it reassuring to know that on Thursday we'll eat 'pasta with sauce and a salad', and that all the ingredients are in the larder. One friend plans menus for a whole month in advance, which I find enormously impressive. She can take full advantage of shopping bargains by buying in bulk when prices are low. Planning ahead saves time and money, and enables you to avoid last-minute dashes to the shops, reducing car use.

KEEPING YOUR SPIRITS HIGH

If, after reading through a few chapters, you are hesitant about getting started on your own green home, even though you see ideas you could use, don't feel guilty and give up. There will be definite reasons for your hesitation.

You may worry about opposition from loved ones. As you get excited about cleaning up your home environment, that enthusiasm may be contagious and your partner or housemates or children may jump on the bandwagon. But they may cling ever more tightly to the remote control device and the microwave instruction booklet, flaunt their drycleaning and throw away the box of used newspaper you were saving for the recycling centre. Don't try to do too much, too soon. Change can be very threatening and you cannot force true cooperation. Be patient – give it time and remember that, no matter how small the beginning, it is always better to do something than to do nothing. If something is worth doing, it is also worth doing a little at a time.

Gradual change is far more likely to be permanent than a crash programme, as anyone who has struggled to lose weight will know. Remember that new ways of doing things soon become old ways. Keep a sense of perspective and don't be hard on yourself when you slip from the straight environmental path. Relish the ironies of life and don't fret when the children regale your mother-in-law with a body count of the wine bottles in the last load you took to the recycling centre. You won't convert anyone to the green cause by being grim and miserable.

Perhaps you are afraid of looking ridiculous riding a bicycle or building a compost heap. Or you may feel you still don't know enough and need more information or advice. Here, the solution is to find other people who share your concerns and want to explore options for change with you. If you are worried about air pollution, increased traffic in your locality or about the pesticides being sprayed along the roadside by the local school, there are certain to be other people worried too. Organizing a food cooperative or joining an allotment society is a way to build a community of people who can share information and practical advice.

You may find yourself depressed at the extent of the problems we face. I've tried to emphasize solutions but environmental issues can be alarming and upsetting. I have faced this myself while writing *The Green Home*, and find that taking action in the world outside my home is essential to maintaining my enthusiasm and hopefulness. Empowerment comes from a sense of hands-on involvement. All of us need to see positive change. If you look around your area you are sure to find good causes vying for your attention, perhaps the conservation of an historical building or building of a wildlife area near a school. Be positive. As well as combating plans to build a shopping centre on a site of specific scientific interest (SSSI), look for projects that will make your part of the world a better place.

There are always trade-offs as we move through our lives with limited time and resources. Pace yourself. Don't try to turn your life upside down and don't feel guilty because you continue to drive your children to their music lessons. Keep looking for options and evaluating your choices. And take time to enjoy and learn about the beautiful world we live in.

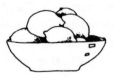

2

WHAT WE SAVE AND SPEND

I used to worry that readers would think an ecology book should concentrate on recycling instead of discussing purchasing habits. Today, green consumerism is an accepted, albeit confusing, trend. But green consumerism has been controversial because it seemed some people were suggesting we could buy our way to a better world. Consumers felt uncertain about all the environmental claims being made for different products. Environmentalists had questions too. Is any product 100 per cent environment-friendly? Isn't consumerism the antithesis of caring for the environment?

While the next chapter concentrates on specific issues for the concerned green shopper, here we will look at our spending, and the flow of money in our society and around the world. We'll also look at how our choices – to live more simply, to invest ethically – can speed solutions to pressing environmental and social problems.

Consumer Society

Economic growth is, according to accepted wisdom, a good and necessary thing. Increasing productivity is a good thing, too, no matter what the human and social cost. We measure standards of living in terms of cars, washing machines and other things we own, without any measure for quality of life. The more people buy – the more the economy grows – the better it is for the country.

Is there an ever-rising standard of living for everyone? Or is there a rising standard of living for some, with corresponding deterioration for others? The notion of limitless growth is a foolish one. All production depends on the input of raw materials which come from the earth; these are in limited supply or replace themselves very slowly. What happens when they run out? It makes no difference whether that happens in 10 years or 1000 – is it appropriate simply to use things up, without ensuring that there is something to take their place?

Do you have a bathroom cabinet full of make-up and different brands of cough syrups or half a dozen different bottles of shampoo? The packages were tempting, you were in a hurry or a friend recommended that new shampoo. Consumption has become a way of life. But do we want to be 'consumers'? Consumers consume – that is, use things up – not a particularly satisfying function for human beings. Most of us would prefer to think that we are acting in the world, affecting other people, creating something of value.

It's natural to want pretty things, and to want new and different things. But the cycle of buy and throw away, buy and throw away has reached dizzying proportions. We felt sick when we read about the hundreds of pairs of shoes Imelda Marcos left behind when she fled the Philippines, but perhaps didn't think so much about just how many pairs are cluttering up our wardrobe. Certainly, there's a big difference between 500 and 15. But where does need turn into desire, and desire turn into greed and dependence?

The problem is simple – we consume too much. Buying green

is not going to affect that (perhaps we will feel so virtuous that we will buy even more!). Neither does green consumerism concern itself with the question of our dependence on a few large firms and the vast multinationals, whose primary interest is corporate profits, not corporate responsibility.

SUSTAINABILITY

In contrast, alternative economists promote the idea of sustainability, which means meeting the needs of the present without compromising the ability of future generations to meet their own needs. It means that no renewable resource (such as timber or clean water) should be used at a rate beyond its capacity to replenish itself and no limited resource (such as coal) should be used up before alternatives are available.

It is difficult for Western politicians to address the problem of consumption squarely, though leaders of developing countries made this an issue at the Rio Earth Summit in 1992 and the Cairo Population Conference in 1994. They prefer to see the reduction of Western consumption only in terms of increasing energy efficiency and better recycling. While this is certainly desirable, the energy used by appliances is often less than the energy used to manufacture and transport them, and the problems of waste cannot be solved by making more efficient refrigerators.

Debate flourishes over the imposition of 'sustainable development' policies through international agreements. Some people claim that poor nations do not have the luxury of richer nations in setting limits on the use of natural resources because of the pressing problems of poverty, and debt repayments to northern leaders. Many say that international agreements forcing poor countries to limit their use of resources will drive them into deeper economic and social turmoil, and that northern countries have unsustainably exploited the resources of their own countries and of the entire world to attain their present high standard of living.

ADVERTISING

It is estimated that the typical consumer receives 5000 advertising messages a day, so many that even the marketing people are worried about overloading the public with advertising clutter. Think of all the adverts you see. Not only those on telly or in magazines: think of the adverts on taxis, T-shirts, even milk cartons. Visible clothing labels and car stickers as well as billboards are forms of advertising. So is a hamburger company's sponsorship of the restoration of an ancient monument. Even in developing countries, walls are plastered with posters advertising soft drinks and cigarettes. Everywhere you turn, somebody is trying to get you to create brand familiarity and persuade you to buy.

Some advertising is informative and necessary. Advertising pays for many of our newspapers, magazines and television programmes. Unfortunately, it also becomes the *raison d'être* for many of them. Most advertising is designed to make you unhappy with what you've got. Our insecurities grease the wheels of commerce.

There is a growing awareness, especially in the US where the problem is most intense, that there need to be restrictions on advertising and on commercialization. In Washington DC, the Center for the Study of Commercialism has promoted, with the help of religious leaders, a coalition to protest about the commercialization of Christmas. They are also organizing campaigns against paid product placements in films, advertising in schools and television advertising aimed at young children.

RETHINKING CONSUMERISM

The first step towards ecologically sound consumption is to think carefully about what you really need and want. Do you think more about what you want to buy than about what you want to do, or be? Are your choices about the future determined by what you own?

There is a growing interest in the new notion of old-fashioned thrift: 'Use it up, wear it out, make it do, or do without' is an old New England saying which was a comfort to many people scaling back their lives in the recession of the early 1990s. Car boot sales in Britain, garage sales in the US, and second-hand or charity shops are doing a booming business.

People are simplifying their lives; choosing simpler homes, simpler meals, simpler clothes, and simpler holidays. This goes with a reconsideration of the things we value, and thought about the limits to our time and energy. The frantic pace of urban life is leading many people, especially parents of young children, to choose to move to smaller towns where they can lead a more balanced life, with time for family, friends and themselves.

Beyond this, environmental and religious organizations are encouraging members to think of 'living simply that others may simply live'. Money and time freed by living more simply are devoted to relief efforts and voluntary work, either locally or in other places where there are special needs.

Since our primary satisfactions in life come from our relationships with our families and friends, the more time we have to enjoy these relationships, and the more our lives are structured to foster stable human connections, the less likely we are to buy compulsively or to buy for status. When a survey found that the Irish had fewer consumer goods than people in other European countries, the Irish were up in arms at the implication that this meant Ireland wasn't as desirable a place to live as Luxembourg. They told interviewers that they were more likely to spend their time arguing about politics or poetry than shopping for a dishwasher.

Maybe if you stop buying so much you'll end up with too much money. But you can give some away or invest it (ethically of course – see below, p. 25). Or you could cut back on the time you spend working, so you have more time for your family, or gardening, or travel – for campaigning on environmental issues or writing that novel you've always talked about.

■Positive Spending

While there is a growing consciousness that there is nothing we can buy that will save the planet, and that we should be looking for ways to reduce overall consumption in our society, humans have for centuries purchased goods and services, and there are ways in which our spending can be a force for good. Economics is crucial to environmental change. Our spending choices have important effects on issues from soil erosion in Norfolk to the destruction of rainforests in Malaysia.

The emphasis in this book is on Britain, but it seems apt to point out certain US economic trends that are likely to occur elsewhere. Americans have, over the past decades, chosen to have a greater number of cheap goods rather than fewer goods of high quality. The result is that they have, as consumers, undermined themselves as producers. When cheapness is the first criterion for shoppers – who would rather consume more than better – jobs are invariably going to move from Lancashire, England – to the Philippines.

Choosing to spend more on a product made closer to home, particularly something well made and durable, is a way to sustain a local economy. In a small town, these choices are clearer. When I stop to buy my milk and biscuits at the little corner grocer, I am helping a shop I value to survive. It really is a matter of survival. Supermarkets (particularly out-of-town ones), and our use of them, have driven small shopkeepers out of business. I like my corner shop, I enjoy the experience of going there and know that its presence makes my locality a better place to live, and I am glad to spend a few pence extra to keep it. In order to preserve strong communities, especially in rural areas, residents need to keep money in the local economy in order to encourage a sufficient diversity of services. This is green consumerism, making sure that the money we spend supports businesses we want and the people who run them.

■The Price of Free Trade

I used to think that I was helping people in Poland or Taiwan by buying things made there. I didn't realize that by buying cheap foreign goods I was encouraging sweatshops, often run by huge international companies. Training shoes are 'made in Taiwan':

uppers sewn in one village, sides in another and a man in a van drives around collecting them for the next stage of manufacture, which takes place entirely in Taiwan. The company whose name goes on the shoe is nothing but a huge marketing department. Workers are paid a dollar a day; the training shoes sell for about £50 a pair. Under current free trade agreements, manual workers in richer countries will continue to lose their jobs (and thus their opportunity to have a lifetime of work and the human dignity that comes from work) to people who will work for less in other parts of the world.

Trade agreements make this kind of production system the way of the future. Opponents of free trade agreements contend that the quality of our food will be eroded as food safety standards are lowered to comply with less stringent international standards. They also contend that local and national decision-making on issues such as genetic engineering will be replaced by unaccountable global processes, and that there will be substantial job losses.

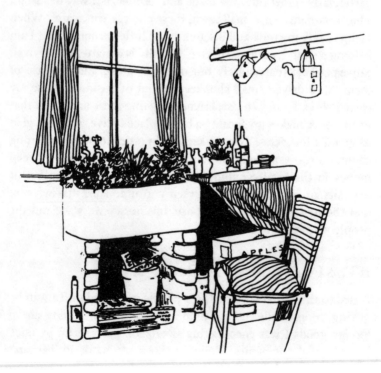

Labour and environmental standards are the major concerns of opponents of trade agreements, but these are complicated issues. To learn more about different views, and about how our shopping choices influence people in other parts of the world, see the Sources at the end of the book. There are schemes run by various organizations and companies to provide people in developing nations with real trade opportunities. Buying from them, buying goods made in Britain and, perhaps most important, buying goods made in your own region are ways you can help to create a healthy economy.

DOES GREEN LIVING COST MORE?

It's unfortunate that many people think green is expensive. When it comes to home ecology, creativity is far more important than cash. People who live on small incomes are, as a rule, easier on the planet than the wealthy. Poorer people necessarily consume less.

Many of the specific tips for ecological homemaking – buying second-hand, refinishing an old chest of drawers, cooking with real potatoes instead of buying oven chips – will save money. Reusing things – from yoghurt cartons (for freezing leftovers) to wine corks (saw in half lengthwise and fix on a leftover board with wood glue to make a practical and charming notice board) – and growing your own fruit and vegetables are excellent ways to keep your expenses down. Basic non-toxic cleaning supplies are very cheap, especially compared with aerosol products.

Some environmental choices will cost more. Organic food from a small farm is more expensive than food grown with chemical pesticides by an international agricultural conglomerate. You may decide that paying more, when your choice means that you are not contributing to pollution or to the exploitation of coffee pickers in the third world, is a fair social contribution. Paying more for better quality products, which will last longer, is ecologically and financially sound. And think in terms of value for money. Orange squash without tartrazine is more expensive than the supermarket brand which contains it, and real orange juice costs more again. But another way of looking at the money question is to ask how much food your money is buying. Orange squash, for example, is sugar, water and flavouring, sometimes with a small proportion of real fruit juice. What about those packets of whipped dessert? They consist of sugar and hydrogenated fat, with a substantial dose of additives and colour.

KEEPING COSTS DOWN

You may be alarmed that many of the foods recommended by environmental and health specialists cost much more than similar items from a supermarket. The extra expense of organically grown food can be compensated for by eating less meat, and cutting out many convenience and snack foods, but it is still important to think about how to obtain good quality food at reasonable prices. People on a low income have far poorer diets, and spend a larger proportion of their income on food, than do people who have more money. Only by making a truly adequate diet (including food free from dangerous additives and pesticides) accessible to everyone, can there be real improvements in the national health.

Organizing a cooperative scheme among a few friends is an easy way to save a great deal of money on food and household supplies like soap and loo paper. Order 'real' meat from a farm and wholefoods (grains, legumes and dried fruits keep for long periods, so you can stock up) in bulk. Contact the Soil Association or the Henry Doubleday Research Association for current listings of organic farms and dairies in your area where you can buy direct. Emphasizing seasonal foods, and letting inexpensive grains, legumes, and vegetables like potatoes and carrots form the mainstays of your diet, keeps basic costs very low and is a healthy way to eat.

■ Creative Acquisition

I once stayed with friends in their tiny New York apartment. They were both designers and wanted their home to demonstrate their talents, but had little money. I was astonished to hear how many of their things had been scavenged from the street – including a pretty chair, several lamps and a rug. It was common for people to put anything they didn't want out on the pavement and a scouting trip early Saturday morning was almost certain to turn up something useful.

Skips are a fabulous source of firewood and scrap timber for building a compost bin, and you can find anything from old bricks to bathtubs in them. I once carpeted a flat with beautiful wool carpet from a skip in front of a Belgrave Square embassy. It needed to be cleaned but was virtually unworn.

Keep your eyes open. My local library replaced its wooden bookcases with adjustable metal shelves a couple of years ago. I talked to the workmen as they were breaking up the old ones and was able to carry home beautiful finished hardwood shelves which would have cost hundreds of pounds.

■Ingenuity

Be creative. Rather than rushing out to buy something new, think about what you might use to do the job and look for new uses for things you might otherwise throw away. For example, plastic trays and cartons make fine drawer dividers. All kinds of containers – from old canning jars to the strange pot Aunt Sophie brought from Mexico – can be used to arrange flowers. Margarine tubs are useful for storing cottons, buttons and beads.

In suggesting this, I do not mean to ignore the way things look and how they perform. Buy beautiful, useful things when you need to. I've found, however, that a more individual style emerges when one applies a little ingenuity to the process of home-making, rather than immediately making a shopping list, and it's possible to save a good deal of money, have a less cluttered home and reduce one's consumption by thinking before getting out the credit cards.

■Pooled Labour and Tools

Building a sense of community, whether a village or a block of flats reduces consumption. People consume more when their lives are very much individualized, where tools and equipment are not shared, where clothes are not passed to younger children in other families, where entertainment has to be purchased. Children need far fewer games and toys when they have many companions. Adults don't rush out to buy things when there are friends and neighbours nearby who can lend a hand or loan a tool (and we need companionship just as much as children do).

Anyone who has seen the Amish barnraising in the film *Witness* will have some idea of the way small rural communities traditionally share labour. No money needs to change hands and the work is a social event which binds the community together. Some version of this is possible even in modern urban neighbourhoods. Why not help a friend draughtproof his house in return for a hand with laying a new floor in your children's playroom? Or have a housewarming and painting party – everybody wears old clothes, and you provide plenty of hot food and cold beer.

■Local exchange trading schemes (LETS)

A growing trend is LETS programmes, a sophisticated form of barter that enables people to make purchases and be paid in turn for their services or products (from calligraphy to cakes) in Olivers (Bath) or Solents (Southampton) rather than in pounds sterling. The concept of LETS developed in Canada in the 1980s and has spread around the world. There are hundreds of local schemes in Britain and the idea is spreading. Records are maintained by a management group, and statements and directories of services are sent out periodically. The scheme benefits people who have skills or products but no job or market outlet within the national economy, and make regions less dependent on outside employment and markets. They also enable people to make greater use of their skills and, naturally, strengthen ties between neighbours. See Sources for more information.

ETHICAL INVESTMENT

If you don't approve of something, you can refuse to buy it and write to the manufacturer to tell them why. You can also encourage good business practice through ethical investing. Conventional investment strategies are based on the assumption that people want maximum returns without regard for social or environmental costs. But an increasing number of investors want to make informed financial decisions, putting their money behind the causes they care about and refusing to endorse corporate irresponsibility. An analysis by *Which?* magazine has found that ethical funds perform overall at least as well as unvetted unit trusts, and there are over 20 ethical and green funds to choose from. A minimum investment is usually £500, and in Britain the total sum invested in ethical funds approaches £1 billion.

Socially responsible investment funds have different criteria, but they generally avoid involvement with companies which are known for environmental problems or violations, produce armaments, tobacco or alcohol, are involved in gambling, pornography, the fur trade, factory farming, animal testing or have links with oppressive regimes. They seek investment in companies with good records in environmental awareness, recycling and waste minimization, pollution control, employee welfare and community involvement.

A related development is the Coalition for Environmentally Responsible Economics (CERES) which drew up a set of corporate principles, first referred to as the Valdez Principles after the oil spill from the *Exxon Valdez* in Alaska, and now called the CERES principles. Close to a hundred corporations – ranging from the Council on Economic Priorities to Ben & Jerry's Ice Cream to General Motors – have signed on, pledging to operate in a way that protects the earth, minimize pollution and waste, conserve energy, offer safe products and services, and use natural resources in a sustainable manner. Its provisions include annual audits of progress and ensuring that at least one board member is qualified to represent environmental interests.

Businesses sometimes seem to take environmental concerns

more seriously than politicians, as they have to think ahead, of future markets, possible lawsuits and ways to strengthen the overall performance of their company. Encourage them to do better by investing in those companies whose performance is good and encourage companies to sign the CERES Principles. If you are ready to invest for good, or want to switch your current investments to an ethical fund, check the most recent *Which?* report and contact one of the umbrella organizations listed in Sources.

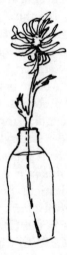

3

BUYING WITH
THE EARTH
IN MIND

A friend of mine was bemused as she looked round her crowd-ed flat, 'How can one person buy this much stuff?' If you are a compulsive consumer, perhaps considering the environmental price-tags, which dangle invisibly from most of the products we buy and use and dispose of, will help you slow down. In Chapter 2 we looked at the way money works in our society and at some of the innovative ways the green homemaker can cut costs. Here, as we consider the decisions we make on the high street or at the shopping centre, is a rundown of environmental problems linked to our shopping choices (environmental price-tags are not writ-ten in pounds and pence, but they can make even cheap items too expensive for the concerned consumer). Then we look at some principles of green shopping and at ways to simplify the shop-ping you do.

To start you off, here is a brief list of the things every green home should have. Further information can be found in the rel-evant chapters:

▶ wholefoods (see Chapter 5);
▶ cloth shopping bags (see Chapter 4);
▶ a bicycle (see Chapter 8);

▶ low energy lightbulbs (see Chapter 14);
▶ clothes drying rack (see Chapter 7);
▶ plants (see Chapter 9).

GLOBAL WARMING

Fossil fuels – coal, oil and natural gas – provide most of the world's commercial energy. Supplies of these are limited (it is estimated that at current rates of use they will be used up in 200 to 300 years, depending on the fuel). When they are burned carbon dioxide (CO_2) is released, and this CO_2 is the primary cause of global warming, the so-called 'greenhouse effect'. The amount of CO_2 in the atmosphere is now more than 15 per cent higher than in pre-industrial times and could easily double within the next 50–100 years. The Meteorological Office has predicted a 5.2°C rise in global temperatures, which would lead to extensive flooding around the world.

Naturally, the price of everything we buy includes a percentage for the energy needed to produce and transport it. As globalization continues and the things we buy come from farther away, energy costs increase. In addition, the chemical-based agriculture that produces most of our food, as well as raw materials for fabrics and many other products, is extremely energy-intensive. Energy is used to produce fertilizers and pesticides, which are often made from petrochemicals, and to manufacture and run mechanical equipment. Large-scale agriculture uses energy for processing, packaging, storage and transportation. The production of cotton, a difficult crop to grow successfully, requires the equivalent of its own weight in oil. Throw in the energy used to get you to the supermarket, and you'll see that our purchases are directly influencing the atmosphere and contributing to global warming. (See Chapter 7 for more on energy.)

THE OZONE LAYER

Only a few years ago substances in aerosol cans, such as hairspray and window cleaners, were routinely combined with the propellant gases called chlorinated fluorocarbons (CFCs) that have been linked to the alarming deterioration of the ozone layer, as well as acting as a potent greenhouse gas. The ozone layer is a sort of light filter for the earth, protecting us from ultra-violet radiation which causes skin cancers and eye problems, and affects human and animal immune systems.

Many manufacturers have responded to scientific and public concern about the ozone layer, and it is now easy to buy aerosols which are 'ozone friendly'. But the ozone layer is still under threat. CFCs and halons are used in rigid and soft foam products (i.e. packaging and insulation as well as foam mattresses and car seats), in commercial and home fridges and freezers, in air conditioners and food industry coolers, in dry cleaning and other solvents, in sterilizing agents and fire extinguishers.

This poses a formidable problem for the foam industry, and they are looking for viable and safe alternatives to CFCs. Manufacturers of air-conditioning equipment are looking for ways to conserve or recycle the CFCs they contain. The Montreal Protocol, agreed in September 1987, states that CFC production must be cut by 35 per cent of the 1986 level by 1999, and manufacturers are scrabbling to find suitable and safe substitutes for ozone-depleting chemicals.

Unfortunately, the substitutes are generally twice as expensive as CFCs. Major developing countries such as China and India did not support the Montreal Protocol because they do not believe that they should be denied the cheap coolants we in the West have used to industrialize. Friends of the Earth has concluded that an immediate 85 per cent reduction in CFCs is necessary to stabilize the ozone damage at its current level and a complete ban on CFCs should be made as soon as possible.

While companies have switched to different propellant gases for aerosols and adopted new labelling, aerosols remain an expensive form of packaging, the very fine particles into which they disperse their contents can be a health threat and they can explode if left next to a source of heat or even in sunlight, posing a hazard to disposal workers. It makes sense to choose an alternative product whenever possible – for example, shaving soap and a brush instead of a can of foam.

PETROCHEMICALS

Toxic waste from the petrochemical industry is a leading source of world pollution, and Barry Commoner, a leading biologist, comments that 'You need to regard the products of the petrochemical industry as evolutionary misfits and therefore very likely to be incompatible with the chemistry of living things. The failure to understand this basic fact has caused the whole problem in chemical pollution. We keep being surprised that chemicals that were perfectly nice and simple to make turn out to have very serious biological consequences.' These environmental consequences include oil spills, air and water pollution from petrol stations, and leachate contamination of groundwater from landfill sites.

Petrochemicals and what is called the commodity chemicals industry developed around the turn of the century, when chemists discovered ways to turn petroleum oil into materials that looked like and could be substituted for more expensive wood, glass, steel and other materials. By the 1950s, the five most important plastics were being made: polyvinyl chloride, polyethylene (in two forms), polypropylene and polystyrene. Chemical companies got bigger and bigger, becoming some of the world's largest corporations. And, since the 1950s, the size of the average chemical plant has increased twentyfold.

Now, however, commodity chemical companies are narrowing their product lines, concentrating on specialized products like paints and acrylics, and moving into other areas, especially pharmaceuticals. Reasons for these changes include the rising cost of environmental regulation and increased competition from developing countries (where regulation is lax).

None the less, petrochemicals surround us. The keyboard I am typing on, the rubber soles on my boots and the switch on my desk lamp are made from plastics. One of the charges levelled at the Body Shop in 1994 was that they used petrochemical ingredients in spite of advertising their products as natural. But most of the products we use every day contain at least some petrochemical product. As a spokesperson from the Body Shop's

Ethical Audit Division pointed out, their staff also use petroleum getting to work each day.

It isn't easy – in fact, it isn't possible at present – to avoid petrochemicals in everyday life. Products made from petroleum resources include plastics, synthetic fibres, newspaper print and a huge array of other common items. Plastics are perhaps the most pernicious. They can be water-resistant, light and almost unbreakable. They are also cheap. The trouble is that they last for ever and, although recycling is possible, in theory it is a long way off in practice for most of the plastic we use. Much packaging is made from layers of different plastics, which cannot be reprocessed in combination. There are also toxicity problems associated with many plastics and dangerous dioxins are given off when they are incinerated.

There are alternatives, however, and people and companies who care about the environment will look for them. Ask your printer about soya-based inks. Choose rattan wastebaskets, paper packaging and natural fibre clothing. While candles provide romantic lighting for dinner parties, they are made from petroleum-derived wax. As an alternative, use more expensive beeswax candles, revive an ancient mode of lighting with an olive oil lamp or make rushlights from native rushes and tallow (see Richard Mabey's *Plants with a Purpose* for instructions).

DISPOSABILITY

All the things we throw away – and should try to recycle – are things we have bought. We buy packaging – the cost of a sturdy cardboard box and polystyrene casing is included in the price you pay for your new home computer – and packaging accounts for approximately 5 per cent of all consumer spending. Of course the computer needs to be packaged, to protect it, but the polystyrene was probably expanded with CFCs and will never be biodegradable. I've spent time on a riverbank clean-up project where crumbled polystyrene and foam peanuts have to be picked out by hand; it is impossible to get every bit and the soil there will forever contain small pieces of foam.

We also pay for disposal. We jointly generate hundreds of thousands of tonnes of rubbish each year. A small proportion of this is burned (creating air pollution) and the remainder goes into landfill sites, in spite of the fact that an estimated 80 per cent could be reused or recycled.

Recycling is better than disposal, but we need to consider how we create so much waste in the first place. More and more of the goods we buy are specifically designed to be used once and thrown away. British Telecom's phonecards are an example: a durable, reusable coin is being replaced by a disposable plastic card packaged in a plastic envelope. Of course customers benefit by having working telephones but the ground is littered with used and broken cards and the plastic envelopes they come in. (It's a small thing, but the concerned consumer uses a coinbox when available and saves the phonecard for emergencies.)

The environmental issues of packaging and disposability include the aesthetics of walking through drifts of rubbish every time we go outside. Do you have to kick your way through a sea of broken hamburger cartons, crisp wrappers and paper cups on your way to catch the bus each morning? Very little of this rubbish could be recycled, even if someone wanted to. The problem isn't restricted to urban areas: walks in the countryside are marred by inescapable and unmistakable signs of the people who have been there before you. Bright purple chocolate bar wrappers and 'disposable' nappies catch the eye, instead of cowslips and hawthorn blossom. Plastic lemonade bottles have eternal life.

CHEMICAL POLLUTION

One of the major environmental debates of the past several years has been over chlorine and chemical compounds called dioxins that are produced by the chlorine bleaching of wood pulp and other industrial processes. Paper bleaching creates dioxins as well as compounds similar to polychlorinated biphenyls, the infamous PCBs which are known to cause sterility and cancer, and which have been associated with the death of seals in the North Sea. Pollution of water around paper mills is an international problem and dioxins are found in bleached paper products, as well as in food and in human tissue.

The Women's Environmental Network (WEN) has campaigned for some years for a reduction in the use of chlorine, especially in paper products such as sanitary towels, disposable nappies and tampons. WEN was successful in 1989 in getting major manufacturers to switch to bleaching processes that do not require chlorine. Unbleached or chlorine-free paper and paper products are now quite common as consumers make their views clear, and as there is increasing evidence of the danger posed by chlorine compounds. Scientist Renate Kroesa, testifying to the Canadian House of Representatives, said: 'Greenpeace will not be convinced that consumers, when made to understand the real tradeoffs between breast milk contamination and the colour of their toilet paper, will not make a wise choice when given one.'

The dispute over chlorine raged for several years, with industry spokespeople insisting that the amounts of dioxin in our environment – produced by incineration, and in the production of paper, plastics and solvents – were harmless. They said placing restrictions on the use of chlorine and chlorine compounds was unreasonable. A Royal Commission on Environmental Pollution recommended increased use of incineration as a way of dealing with the growing waste problem.

In 1994, however, a long awaited US Environmental Protection Agency report on dioxin appeared, substantiating the claims made by environmentalists. The 2000 page study found that dioxins not only cause cancer but have subtle effects on foetal development and the human immune system, even at extremely low levels. The dioxins found in human fatty tissue come from meat, fish and dairy products, which in turn contain dioxins from air and land contamination, mostly, it is thought, from incineration of waste. The only way to reduce human exposure is to reduce the total dioxin load in our environment, and the US government plans to develop a national strategy for reducing or prohibiting the use of chlorine and containing chlorinated compounds. See Chapter 4 (non-disposables, p. 59) and Chapter 12 for what you can do about chemical pollution.

ETHICAL ISSUES

Many of the things offered in our shops come from countries with oppressive regimes, such as China, or where production is causing ecological degradation or economic hardship. Other products have been tested on animals.

Countries which could easily produce enough food to feed their own population instead grow crops for sale to richer nations in order to pay off high interest bank loans (often taken in order to finance expensive and inappropriate Western technology). These problems are complex, related to political and land issues in producer countries and to the hold multinational companies have on third world economies.

Buy what you can from companies or organizations which promote equitable and conscientious development. Traidcraft, for example, sells a wide range of household goods, clothes, tea and coffee from the third world, and ensures that the producers themselves receive a fair price for their goods. The Body Shop has a growing Trade Not Aid programme, and many other companies are looking for ways to support ethical international trade.

GREEN PRODUCTS ARE:

- made from natural, non-toxic materials;
- energy efficient;
- recycled and/or recyclable;
- unbleached or chlorine-free;
- simply packaged;
- durable and sometimes reusable;
- easy to repair;
- produced without cruelty to animals;
- made and sold locally whenever possible.

Responsible meat eating is discussed in Chapter 5. The green homemaker will want to avoid meat which has been raised by intensive farming methods, as well as cosmetics and toiletries tested on animals. There are considerable concerns about the way in which animals are kept, and slaughtered, which must influence our approach to meat-eating. Transport of live animals abroad is also an issue that many of us are disturbed about. Vegetarians and vegans may want to avoid products that contain animal ingredients.

SHOPPING CLOSE TO HOME

You've read about the demise of the corner shop and seen old favourites close down or move away. Shopping centres are increasingly taking shopping away from our homes into centralized sites which are geared to car owners. Many of us use local shops only for spur-of-the-moment purchases, like a pint of milk or packet of butter. Local shops are often more expensive, with less selection than the megastores. The much vaunted choice we are offered in big stores is, however, misleading (aren't things often much of a muchness?), and in any case dazzling variety is a spur to over-consumption. Small shops will give individual attention and can often obtain special goods for you if you ask. But doing your shopping near home saves time, transportation costs and fuel. By keeping your neighbours in business you enrich your own locality.

Architects at the Center for Environmental Structure in Berkeley, California, write: 'we believe that people are not only willing to walk to their local corner groceries, but that the corner grocery plays an essential role in any healthy neighborhood: partly because it is more convenient for individuals; partly because it helps to integrate the neighborhood as a whole.' In fact, local shops are one of the most important elements in our perception of an area as a community.

Of course you are not going to give up your weekly supermarket shop immediately, especially when you are not sure what the alternatives are. Such changes have to be gradual. Over the past couple of years I have found my supermarket shopping lists growing shorter and shorter as I find other places and other ways to stock my home and kitchen.

THINGS THAT LAST

Think about durability and repairability when you shop. Buying higher quality and more costly items is an incentive to choose carefully and to make things last. A fountain pen will outlast dozens of plastic biros and is a pleasure to write with. A good one will last a lifetime. (If you cannot trust yourself not to lose an expensive pen, be frugal with ordinary plastic pens and biros, and use refills.)

Most ordinary household mugs and glasses are easy to break, and you'll get better wear by buying things designed for restaurant and hotel use. These range from the simple and serviceable to the elegant. Look in catering shops, which are also a source of heavy cooking pans and utensils.

A really good piece of clothing might last 50 years. This may sound crazy in these days of cheap and cheerful high street fashion, and ever-changing fashion silhouettes, but quite a few of us have a 'vintage' tweed jacket or a Victorian nightdress among our clothes. Furniture, assuming that it is well made in the first place, can last for centuries.

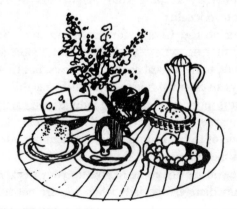

LOCAL PRODUCTS

John Seymour, the grandfather of sustainable living, once wrote: 'Slowly and steadily, I am ridding my home, as far as I can, of mass-produced rubbish, and either learning to do without certain things or replacing them with articles made out of honest materials by people who enjoyed making them and who, by long diligence and training, have qualified themselves to make them superbly.' This is a constructive approach which we can all adopt.

There are hundreds of small businesses and craftspeople around the UK, and abroad, who sell their goods direct to callers as well as by mail order. Scottish tweeds, hand made wooden toys, wrought iron kitchenware and smoked salmon from the Outer Hebrides are only a few of the many things available. Prices are relatively low because there are no middlemen, and it is satisfying to know that your money is going to the person who has actually made the thing you are going to use. The human contact is delightful and you won't find yourself wearing the same sweater as a quarter of a million other people.

Try to buy from small farms and cottage industries. A demand for real ale has put small brewers back in business and a demand for real British food is encouraging many small producers into the market. T. S. Eliot, who was a great cheese fan, mourned the demise of traditional British cheese some 40 years ago. He would be delighted to see that it is back in the news and on our plates. Ask around – there may be a potter who lives down the road or a skilled seamstress a few doors away. Use a local joiner instead of going to a large building contractor and buy prepared food for a party from a local vegetarian caterer instead of from a big chain store.

OLD THINGS

Buying things second-hand is a way to save money as you recycle. There are second-hand or 'nearly new' shops in many towns which sell good quality clothing, with the shop taking a percentage of the sale price. Some sell very expensive designer garments at a considerable reduction. For household items there are auctions and salerooms, ranging from cheap and seedy to very exalted indeed. Good quality second-hand furniture is often a far better buy than new items and a reconditioned vacuum cleaner may give many more years of service than a bright new plastic one.

The quality and range of second-hand clothes varies considerably. It's worth getting to know the good shops and popping in regularly to look at their new stock. 'Vintage' clothes which sell at high prices at trendy market stalls can sometimes be found for next to nothing at jumble sales, where some stallholders do much of their buying. Factory seconds are sometimes available direct and are found everywhere during annual sales. In fact, buying goods with slight flaws – including oddly shaped eggs from a local farm – is good domestic management and makes ecological sense.

Jumble and car boot sales have the lowest prices. The best jumble sales are at churches and schools in prosperous areas, and there is likely to be a fierce queue ready long before the doors open. Take your own bags and small change, and be ready for a fight to get to the tables. Jumble sale helpers are likely to get first chance at the better articles, something to consider when you are asked to lend a hand.

Remember that charity shops do not exist to give you a bargain but to raise money for the organization's projects. (Prices, however, vary a great deal. While an Oxfam shop in the country might charge 50p for a skirt, a similar garment might sell for £5 in central London due to higher rents and rates.)

'Surplus' stores are full of peculiar and sometimes useful things. I've bought heavy ex-army cotton sheets, excellent for tablecloths, napkins and curtain lining. Or you could check the advertisements in newsagents' windows and local papers. Better still place your own, asking for the things you want. Some people barter something they want to get rid of for something they want.

Paying For Labour

In ecological terms, it makes sense to do certain jobs in a labour-intensive way: hand-weeding, for example, rather than using herbicides. There are times when it is possible to employ someone to do a task which would otherwise require some heavy, noisy, expensive and polluting piece of equipment: raking leaves in autumn, for example, rather than hiring a leaf blower. The ecological choice is to use human labour and create local employment.

Sympathetic Materials

While plastics last virtually for ever, cluttering up the planet, natural materials like paper, cloth, wood and fur will disappear into the soil in a year or so, and actually enrich it. To see this, bury a variety of household items in your compost heap or in a deserted patch of ground: a milk bottle top, an old beach shoe, a piece of cellophane wrapping, a cereal box and plastic liner, a worn out polycotton shirt, a glass jar and a tin can. Which will disappear first? Which items will outlive you and your grandchildren? If you choose natural materials – sisal door mats, a wooden file box, leather shoes – they will not pollute the earth long after you've left it. And by choosing materials which come from the earth, we also become more conscious of our connections with it and more appreciative in our use.

Promoting Biodiversity

At the Rio Earth Summit in 1992, governments negotiated a Convention on Biological Diversity – or biodiversity, a term meaning the earth's ecosystems, species and genetic resources. The UN's Environment Programme is also secretariat for biodiversity-related conventions such as the Convention on International Trade in Endangered Species of Wild Fauna and

Flora (known, thank goodness, as CITES). The latter convention aims to control trade in endangered species, ranging from ivory to rhinoceros horns to seal penises.

But the loss of species comes much closer to home. We are losing apple orchards at an alarming rate, though in Britain they have been one of the most important wildlife habitat areas in populated areas for centuries. There used to be over 6000 varieties of apple in Britain, favourites in each region. Now, shops sell only two or three varieties, most from abroad.

Why does biodiversity matter? The earth consists of hundreds of thousands of overlapping areas in which complex relationships between animals, plants, insects and microbacteria form ecosystems, each with an equilibrium that has developed over hundreds of thousands of years. Human influences have altered these delicately poised systems so dramatically in the recent past that species are disappearing with consequences we cannot foretell.

Harvard biologist E. O. Wilson calls the earth 'an intricate tapestry of interwoven life forms'. He estimates that 50,000 species are condemned to extinction each year (almost entirely as the result of human activity, such as logging) in the tropical rainforests, where there is a greater density of species than anywhere else on earth and where some of the most prized medicines of the modern era have been discovered.

To encourage biodiversity we should leave existing ecosystems and wild places alone, concentrating new buildings on land that is already disturbed, and we should provide wildlife spaces in our gardens and neighbourhoods.

Your shopping can promote biodiversity. Here are some ideas.

▶ Refuse to buy rainforest hardwoods.

▶ Choose woods from a variety of native European species: beech, oak, ash.

▶ Buy a variety of foods: white as well as brown eggs (they come from different types of chicken), old varieties of apple and potato, multigrain bread.

▶ In your garden, plant old roses and open-pollinated (non-hybridized) seeds.

▶ Eat wild plants such as dandelion and nettle, blackberries and elderberries, and make traditional hedgerow drinks like sloe gin.

▶ Let manufacturers know that you want products made from more species: paper, for example, made from hemp or jute or water hyacinth.

▶ Buy recycled paper to discourage the clearcutting of forests and single-crop forestry.

BOYCOTTS

The avoidance of certain types of food or the products of particular countries or companies is a powerful consumer tool. The success of a widespread boycott of tuna fish resulted in dramatic changes in the fishing industry in the late 1980s. It is impossible to give a list of things to boycott, but a few examples are campaigns asking that shoppers avoid buying pencils made by certain companies using jelutong, an endangered rainforest wood, and cosmetics from companies that use animal testing. Christian Aid has run a campaign to pressure the Colombian flower industry to reduce pesticide use and improve working conditions – after The Netherlands, Colombia is Britain's second largest supplier of flowers. In the Sources you will find several journals that list current boycotts. The most notable campaign is the long-standing protest against Nestlé milk products in the third world.

Susan George, a respected researcher on international food issues, has suggested a boycott of products from 'corporate junk-food mongers' – makers of soft drinks and sugary cereal flakes, for example – because these companies aggravate malnutrition in the third world by promoting their nutritionally marginal products as alternatives to indigenous staple foods. The same could be said of junk-food promotion in Britain.

SHOPPING SIMPLIFIED

Green shopping may take a bit longer as you buy less at the supermarket and more from other sources, but you will probably find yourself spending less time in the long run. I am sympathetic to the harried Saturday shopper who gets frustrated with the local high street – it's almost impossible to park and you're buying too much to carry home on foot – but I still believe we should support local shopping because in the long term those shops, and the locality they create, will determine the social characteristics of the places we live in. Community groups need to join forces with small shopkeepers to help them provide the products and services we want.

Organization makes an enormous difference and your shopping time should be much more enjoyable. Here are some tips.

▶ Stock up as much as your budget and cupboard space allow. Whole grains and legumes, toilet paper and cleaning products can be bought in bulk and last virtually for ever. Stocking up not only saves money and the hassle of running out in the middle of the holidays, but eliminates a considerable amount of packaging.

▶ Keep track of things you are running low on by ensuring that there is a pad of paper and a pencil in the kitchen and the bathroom. Everyone in the household should learn to add to these lists.

▶ Make out a shopping checklist of everything you normally keep on hand, arranged into categories by shop or even by aisle. Make photocopies and tick off the things you need.

▶ Shop in the same shops regularly – you'll sometimes get better service and knowing the layout speeds up shopping considerably.

▶ Stock up on gifts, if your budget allows, so you don't have to make a special trip to get a gift for a mid-week birthday party.

▶ Make shopping enjoyable by combining it with outings, and by visiting small producers and craftspeople.

4

THE THREE RS: REDUCE, REUSE, RECYCLE

In the early 1970s, when my father was making ecology runs into the California foothills, recycling was a virtuous activity adopted by a few eager souls. Today it has become part of our daily lives, an economic necessity and a civic virtue.

Recycling generally means the reprocessing of an industrially produced material like glass or metal. But a more cost-effective form of recycling is to reuse things. Containers can and should be designed for reuse. The most obvious example is the British milk bottle: each pinta is filled an average of 12 times. I grew up in the United States where most milk delivery disappeared in the '60s. None the less, long dusty summers at my grandparents' home in Iowa always included daily trips to the store for icy bottles of soda, which we financed by combing the roadsides for discarded bottles. My father's ecology collections included the drink cans that had by then replaced glass bottles, along with the dangerous metal tabs which littered roadsides.

Recycling continues to be high on the environmental agenda and bottle banks are increasingly common. Critics, however, contend that the emphasis on recycling draws attention from the more significant steps we should be taking: reducing packaging and switching to reuse systems such as bottle refilling. And stories continue to surface about the inability of industry to cope with the quantities of glass and paper available for recycling.

OUR WORLD OF WASTE

Recycling and reuse has always been part of local economies, and only during the past few decades have we ignored the resource potential in things we no longer need. Overflowing bins and a growing waste problem are the result, with black bags piled along city streets and litter festooning country hedgerows.

In the past, everything was put to good use. Much great country cooking is the result of our grandmothers' determination to waste nothing and recycling has always been a natural part of household management. And times are changing, with much talk about the three Rs: reduce, reuse and recycle. Behind this change is an increased awareness of the environmental consequences of waste. There have been explosions of methane gas which has leaked from landfill tips, and methane is a potent contributor to global warming. Toxic leachate fluid seeping from a tip can contaminate groundwater.

As a result of these factors and the increased distance rubbish has to be transported from urban regions, rubbish collection and landfill costs are rising dramatically. Economic pressures are combining with environmental concerns to encourage new approaches.

Most environmental specialists as well as consumer groups believe that a greater effort should be put into reducing the amount of domestic waste, by forcing manufacturers to reduce packaging, by developing refill systems (this is sometimes called 'precycling') and by developing local composting schemes for the 20 per cent of domestic waste that is made of biodegradable vegetable material.

Incineration used to be considered an environmentally sound way to get rid of garbage, as well as a potentially useful source of heat and energy. But it has become a nightmare problem for many communities, especially as new research on dioxin and other chemical hazards show the danger presented by even well-managed incineration facilities. In fact, says the *Ecologist* magazine, 'the better the air pollution control, the more toxic the ash'.

Part of the appeal of incineration was that it did not require a shift in patterns of consumer behaviour or business practice. While incineration continues to take place, public attitudes and recent research findings have pushed policy makers towards other solutions to the waste crisis.

WHOSE BACKYARD?

When there was plenty of landfill space and little publicity about leakage of toxic chemicals, we were able to ignore the waste we produced. But times have changed. We can no longer afford to be squeamish. While rubbish doesn't sound as important as education or law enforcement, next to these it is the most expensive item in many local government budgets.

As cheap, accessible landfill sites fill up, rich countries are sending their waste abroad and poor countries have accepted not only domestic rubbish but also toxic waste, in spite of the long-term risks to their own citizens. Greenpeace has estimated that over 10 million tons of waste have been exported to Eastern Europe and developing countries since 1986.

None of us wants this rubbish in our backyard, but everywhere is someone's backyard. There are obvious ethical questions raised by the prospect of American rubbish being buried in Cornish tin mines or West German industrial waste in Northern Cyprus, but also by London's waste being buried in landfill sites in Hertfordshire and Essex. Throughout the world, waste sites and incinerators are frequently sited in poorer areas, often those with large ethnic minority populations. They are placed in these areas because richer ones have the political clout and organization resources to fight a NIMBY (not in my back yard) battle. Companies choose a place where resistance will be weak, where people may even be swayed by a few token jobs for local residents. There is a growing movement for environmental justice, demanding non-discriminatory policies and full legal recourse for any area suggested as a possible waste site.

REDUCE

To reduce the total amount of waste we produce we need to rethink our buying and particularly the way we expect goods to be packaged. Become a canny shopper. Try not to buy things you don't need or want. If you're not sure, try a sample or buy a small size, or go away and think about the purchase for a couple of days, particularly if it is a major one. In Chapter 2 you will find plenty of information about reducing consumption in general, so here we'll look at some special problems.

■Packaging

Next time you unload your weekly shopping, take a good look at how much packaging there is: cardboard boxes, plastic and styrofoam trays, plastic film, plastic bags, foil packages, tin cans, aluminium cans, plastic and glass bottles. Start counting layers when you are next out shopping. Microwave meals are infamous: a microwavable soup–and–sandwich snack which won Package of the Year award from a packaging industry magazine has six separate layers of packaging, five of them plastic.

Organic food at the supermarket seems to be packaged even more than 'conventional' produce – organic swedes, for example, are wrapped in clingfilm to differentiate them from chemically-grown produce.

The packaging industry uses 39 million tonnes of materials each year, for which we pay £5000 million. This is no paltry sum we're talking about – remember, you bought the package too! Packaging performs a number of functions. It protects the product during transport and storage; keeps it dry; enables it to be boxed or stacked neatly; displays it to advantage; makes it easy to carry or easy to use; and carries information. But packaging is also used as an advertising medium and as a way to increase the prominence of items on display.

What makes for 'sympathetic' packaging? The minimum necessary to protect the goods inside, it should be reusable, recyclable or biodegradable.

An old stock-in-trade direct action technique is to leave any unnecessary packaging at the check-out. You could bring a letter with you explaining why you are refusing the packaging. Don't lumber the till operator with a bunch of bags – ask for the manager. This will be more effective if a group of people do it together, perhaps to accompany a day of action outside local shops. The Women's Environmental Network has run a 'Wrap It Up' campaign with 'Send It Back' labels to be used to post superfluous packaging back to manufacturers or shops, challenging them to justify anything excessive or inappropriate – contact them for more information and action packs.

TO REDUCE PACKAGING:

- buy in bulk and in the largest container you can manage;
- cut down on canned and bottled food;
- buy in returnable/refillable containers;
- choose products such as laundry liquid packed in bags or refill packs;
- look for concentrated products;
- avoid 'mixed' packaging (e.g. juice boxes, aerosols and bubble packs);
- buy loose items;
- choose paper wrapping in preference to plastic;
- carry your own shopping bags or use the shop's own boxes.

■Disposables

Many common household articles have been specifically designed to be disposable. These are usually made from paper or plastic, placing unnecessarily heavy demands on natural wood and oil resources. There are times when modern disposables are very handy, but the following alternatives are better for the environment.

Paper towels

Use terry towels for your hands and a dishcloth for the worktop
or spills. Drain fried food on brown paper bags saved from the
greengrocer's or on opened cardboard egg cartons.

Sponges

Cotton dishcloths last much longer than synthetic sponges. Real
cellulose sponges are a biodegradable choice.

Cleaning cloths

Accumulate a good supply of cotton cleaning rags, cut from old
sheets or old clothes. (If you are short of old sheets, buy some for
50p at a jumble sale.) Linen is good for windows. Make your own
cleaning cloths by folding an 18 x 18 in square of cotton terry in
half and sewing up the long side to form a tube. All the edges will
need to be hemmed, unless you start with outgrown terry nappies. Refold the cloth and use both sides, then turn inside out for
another four fresh surfaces.

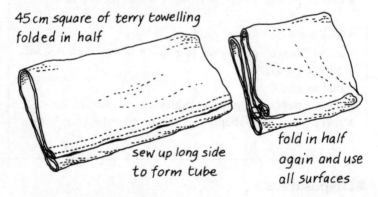

45 cm square of terry towelling
folded in half

sew up long side
to form tube

fold in half
again and use
all surfaces

Homemade cleaning cloths

Paper napkins

Cloth napkins are efficient and far nicer to use than paper napkins. For every day, choose a sturdy cotton fabric which does not
need to be ironed. Many ready-made napkins are made of synthetics (useless on sticky fingers) or linen (too much trouble for

daily use), so you may want to buy a suitable fabric and make your own. Terry works well. A good short-cut is to buy textured cotton tea towels in a suitable pattern, cut them in half and hem the cut edge.

A personalized napkin ring for each family member saves washing – when the napkin is still clean, tuck it back into the ring and put it aside for the next meal. Plain wooden rings or curtain rings can be painted, and gluing on seashells is an attractive way to decorate them.

Food storage bags, aluminium foil and plastic film

Buy reusable plastic or glass containers with lids, or use a plate as a cover. Rather than cover baking dishes with foil, use an upended pie plate or baking tray. Vegetables keep best if wrapped in a damp tea towel, not plastic, and use cloth vegetable bags. Use waxed paper linings from breakfast cereal boxes for wrapping sandwiches. Paper bags from the greengrocer's can replace paper towels for draining fried food.

Sturdy plastic bags can be washed and used many times. Stick them over an empty wine bottle or a whisk in your drainer to dry, or make a simple rack to dry them on.

Labelled yoghurt cups and other plastic containers can be used for storage and freezing.

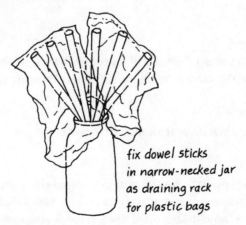

fix dowel sticks
in narrow-necked jar
as draining rack
for plastic bags

Plastic bag dryer

Coffee filters and tea bags

Use a percolator or a cafetière, and loose tea instead of individually wrapped teabags. Instant coffee is not the answer because it is hugely wasteful of energy.

Paper and polystyrene cups and paper plates

Real dishes are so much more pleasant to use. Keep a set of old dishes for use in the garden or on picnics, and if you travel by car, keep several mugs and some cutlery in a basket, ready for impromptu picnics. I take my own coffee mug or a small flask into fast-food places along the motorway.

Bin liners

Line bins with sheets of newspaper, or those plastic carrier bags you can't bring yourself to throw away. Most of your rubbish will be dry if you compost food scraps.

Carrier bags

You can buy durable canvas shopping bags. String bags are great to tuck into a handbag or pocket.

Nappies

For lots about switching to cloth nappies, turn to Chapter 16, p 266.

Baby wipes

Some tissues and a flannel will do the trick most of the time, and you'll avoid the various 'medicated' cleaners these are saturated in.

Facial tissues

Cotton handkerchiefs are a nice alternative.

Razors

Disposable plastic razors are astonishingly cheap, but an appalling waste of raw materials. While you might consider switching to an old-fashioned open razor, a reasonable compromise is to use a razor for which you only need to buy refill blades.

Sanitary products and toiletries

When you buy supplies like cotton wool, cotton buds and tampons, look for those made from biodegradable materials: cardboard and 100 per cent cotton. (The presence of synthetic fibres in tampons increases the growth rate of the bacteria which causes Toxic Shock Syndrome – another good reason for choosing cotton.) As unbleached products become available, buy them. And contact the Women's Environmental Network for more information on the health and environmental problems associated with the use of tampons and disposable sanitary towels.

Tights

Some 500 million pairs of tights and stockings are sold each year in the UK – 23 pairs for each woman in the country. Since this is a 'disposable' article of clothing, you might think about going barelegged when possible, wearing socks or switching to sturdy cotton tights.

Batteries

Batteries contain a wide variety of toxic substances, including zinc, mercuric chloride, lead and cadmium, and manufacturing them takes 50 times more energy than they produce. Choose equipment and toys than can run on mains power, and save up for rechargeable batteries and a charger (far cheaper in the long run).

REUSE

The kind of reuse discussed above – refill systems, for example – are not the only ways to give the things we use and buy a longer life. Creative reuse within the home is a way to reduce expenses as well as waste. You can also buy and restore old items, and repair worn articles of clothing and pieces of furniture. Professional repair services are more difficult to find than they used to be, and it is often more expensive to have mass-produced goods repaired than to buy new ones. The shoddy impermanence of much of what we buy makes it difficult to maintain things through a lifetime.

A big part of the problem is that so much of what we can buy is of such poor quality that in a couple of months a new pair of shoes is looking shabby and down at the heel. And they often aren't made of materials that can be touched up and repaired. Who could repair them anyway – and wouldn't you be told that they aren't worth mending?

There's a curious contradiction here: good quality, expensive items (from shoes to umbrellas to shaving brushes) tend to be made of natural materials which, when they do eventually find their way into the rubbish, will gently break down and disappear, while cheap items which will only last, at best, a couple of years are made of synthetic materials which will not.

■Repairs

A cook's spoon, a carpenter's hammer and a gardener's trowel are essential tools, as is the word processor I've used to write this book. Tools help us to accomplish and create, but most of us are pretty feeble when it comes to looking after them. Think how you envy people who are good with their hands and how much in demand a handy man or woman is. And think of the amounts of money we pay to have our machines serviced.

Mechanical ineptitude leads to a great deal of waste. Learn to love your tools and take care of them. Buy things that can be repaired and for which you can buy replacement parts. Ask about servicing when you buy.

Buy sturdy, well-made tools and keep them in good condition. Read the instructions. They may not be very inspiring pieces of literature, but it's well worth coming to grips with their terminology and structure.

Before calling for help, make an effort to solve the problem yourself. Don't be intimidated by dials and lights; try to think of reasons for the problem. Assemble a reference shelf: a folder with all the instruction leaflets for appliances and electronic equipment, as well as basic books. The Reader's Digest guides are good, and I collect old repair manuals to help me repair second-hand purchases like my faithful 1950s toaster.

And read *Zen and the Art of Motorcycle Maintenance*, by Robert Pirsig, if you want to explore the subject of mechanical repair in exquisite detail.

■Donations

Many charitable organizations and voluntary groups welcome donations of clothes, books and miscellaneous articles, which they resell to raise money.

Telephone charity stores to find out when they accept donations. Some groups will collect larger items from your home.

Ensure that anything you pass on is clean and still useful. Really worn clothing is better turned into dust cloths.

Pin sets of clothing and bag articles which should stay together. Do not remove buttons! Attach a note to old appliances or electronic equipment to say that it works or needs certain repairs.

Save household items such as yoghurt cups and egg cartons for schools and playgroups.

Be creative: our local doctors' surgery was delighted with a large bundle of fairly current magazines.

Enquire before making donations. For example, disaster appeals do not normally take used clothing, because it would need to be fumigated and is often inappropriate for the countries in need.

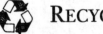 RECYCLING

At last we reach the third R, recycle. If you have simplified your life (Chapter 1), reduced your overall consumption (Chapter 2), bought simply packaged products and bought in bulk (Chapter 3), recycling won't be a major enterprise.

First, find out what the recycling facilities are in your area by telephoning the council – remember, every telephone call about recycling will emphasize its importance. Also contact Friends of the Earth and ask to be put in touch with your local group, who should be able to tell you about Scout groups wanting newspapers or shops wanting carrier bags. A growing number of communities are offering kerbside recycling, often by popular demand, but the economic margins are tight and depend on stable prices for recycled materials.

Second, work out a neat, convenient system for sorting types of waste. Separation of different types of waste is crucial to any recycling programme, whether in your home or nationwide. Once you get used to recycling, the idea of tossing everything into the same container will seem messy and unpleasant. And when you see how vigorously your garden grows with compost made from vegetable scraps, you won't dream of dropping coffee grounds into the same container as newspapers and last night's wine bottle.

Third, arrange things so that you can separate and store everything, except perhaps bulky newspapers, in one spot. Under the kitchen sink is a central place in many homes, but you may find a utility room or back porch more convenient. David Goldbeck, an American kitchen designer, suggests swinging cupboard doors with a 6–9 in gap at the top. These block the bins from view but

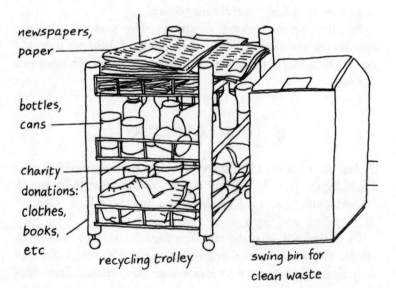

newspapers, paper

bottles, cans

charity donations: clothes, books, etc

recycling trolley

swing bin for clean waste

Recycling corner

allow a busy cook to throw a rinsed vinegar bottle into the right bin. A container which can be opened with your foot is good too, though most such bins are too small for a family's waste.

RECYCLING TIPS

• Make your system attractive, a permanent part of your kitchen. A sturdy pine crate or a children's plastic toybox will last a long time.

• Choose containers based on the recycling available in your area and how you'll be transporting the materials.

• Use bins or boxes, not plastic bags. You can't see what's in a bag and they flop.

• Use the largest containers that space allows and you can carry. You shouldn't have to move or empty a bin, except for kitchen waste, more than once a week.

• Choose containers which are easy to carry, empty and clean. This is especially important with wet waste and heavy glass.

• Place the containers as near as possible to site of use. Most recyclables should be stored, at least temporarily, in the kitchen. You may want to put a big bin (or an attractive basket) for newspapers in the sitting room.

• Take up as little floor space as possible, with stackable bins or boxes on shelves, but ensure that every bin is in position for a quick toss.

• Label containers to make sorting easy for your family and guests (use cut-out magazine illustrations to help small children).

• Include a space for items you intend to donate.

■Recycling Simplified

Certain simple choices will make recycling considerably less effort.

▶ Eat more simply, using bulk purchased foods, and avoiding packaged meals and takeaways (see Chapter 5).

▶ Make water your drink of choice and use a filter rather than purchasing bottled water.

▶ Eliminate as much junk mail as possible.

▶ Cut your magazine and newspaper subscriptions to the bone.

▶ Unclutter your home.

■Recycling Summary

Paper

Can be recycled and small amounts can go into the compost heap. Newspapers can also be used as a mulch (see Chapter 15). Tie newspapers into bundles with natural fibre string, or pack them in paper bags or cardboard boxes.

Glass

A painless way to clean bottles for the recycling centre (if they contained something messy, which could smell) is to fill them with warm soapy water from your washing-up water and leave them overnight. Pour out half the water, put the lid back on, give it a good shake and rinse. With bottles for recycling, throw lids away and remove any metal or plastic; paper labels are OK.

Glass jars are excellent for pantry storage, as well as for jam and pickle making. Large jars make permanent containers for flour and grains and beans; they look nice and are easier to cope with than plastic bags.

Aluminium

Although we use over 4 billion aluminium drinks cans in the UK each year, less than 10 per cent are recycled. Recycling not only saves 95 per cent of the energy needed to produce aluminium but reduces the amount of land, often in tropical rainforests, being destroyed to mine the bauxite ore it comes from. Drink cans, aluminium foil, trays and pie plates can all be washed and taken to your nearest recycling centre. Large aluminium items, like window frames, can be recycled, too.

Steel cans

These are harder to recycle because they contain several metals that have to be separated, but steel cans can be sorted from other rubbish with a magnet. It's worth recycling both aluminium and steel, says *Which?* magazine, but it's far more important to reduce the number of cans you buy.

Plastics

These have generally gone to landfill sites, as recycling programmes are few and far between. This is changing rapidly, however, with the launch of new fabrics and several ranges of outdoor clothing, and gear such as sleeping bags made from recycled PET (polyester terephthalate) plastic, the hard plastic in which many kinds of soft drinks are now sold, along with boots and shoes with soles made from recycled rubber tyres.

Environmentalists agree that recycling is far more important than the development of so-called 'biodegradable' plastics and you can help create a market by purchasing products made from recycled materials. Don't burn plastics, as the smoke they give off is often toxic. Plastic pump-top and spray bottles are useful for home-made cleaners or for repackaging products bought in large containers, and yoghurt pots can be used as lunch containers.

Food scraps

Vegetable and fruit trimmings and leftover food of all kinds can be composted into a fine and nourishing fertilizer. You can include everything from sandwich crusts to nut shells; the only things to avoid are citrus rinds, which break down slowly, and meat scraps, which can attract vermin. (Leftover fat won't compost well but it can be mixed with seed or stale bread crumbs to attract birds to your garden.) Grass clippings and autumn leaves can be added, too, and I include small amounts of paper, matchsticks, and cotton wool – anything that will break down naturally.

It's estimated that 20 per cent of household waste is compostable, so some councils are establishing programmes to encourage residents to compost their food scraps as a substantial contribution towards meeting the EU's legislative target for reducing household rubbish by 25 per cent by the year 2000. You can help to make this happen; see below for tips about efficient composting.

■ Composting Tips

Use a galvanized metal or stainless steel container, as it can be sterilized with boiling water and won't hold smells like plastic. Line it with newspaper for easy emptying.

Spread a piece of newspaper before you start chopping raw food. When you have finished, gather up the edges and put the whole thing in the compost bin.

Try composting with worms, as many residents in the London Borough of Sutton have. It may sound strange but the bins are compact and efficient, and great fun for children. I look forward to the day when they are as ubiquitous as microwaves. Properly

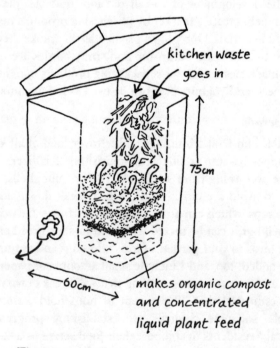

kitchen waste goes in

75cm

60cm

makes organic compost and concentrated liquid plant feed

The wormery

managed, the bins do not smell because the garbage is digested before it can rot. They can be kept inside or out, and the end result is a rich black material which can be used in the garden or for potted plants. See Sources for more information.

If you're planning a new kitchen, have a hole cut in your work-top, covered with a pivoted cutting board, through which vegetable trimmings can be pushed into a concealed bin.

Or fit the top drawer under your worktop with a restaurant-size stainless steel pan. Peelings can be pushed into the drawer, and the stainless steel is easy to clean and does not hold odours.

■Hazardous Waste

Toxic wastes, including used batteries, old paint and paint thinners, need particularly thoughtful disposal. Councils should provide a separate collection point for hazardous materials. Do not allow them to enter the water system; seal them and put them into the collection bin for landfill disposal. Used motor oil can be recycled and should be taken to a garage which collects it. Some garages collect used oil and anti-freeze for reprocessing. Some communities are starting paint exchanges so DIY materials can be made full use of.

Another thing to think of when throwing rubbish away is the potential danger to wildlife. Animals can be caught in plastic netting and deer have been known to die as a result of swallowing plastic bags. The plastic rings which hold packs of beer and soft drinks cans together can be lethal too. When spending a day outdoors, take your rubbish home with you!

■The Paper Problem

We are profligate with paper, so accustomed to an endless supply of beautiful white writing surfaces as well as books and newspapers that we forget that in most of the world paper is a precious commodity. A typesetter from Prague told me that he would never dream of running off three copies of a manuscript or making triple copies of routine correspondence.

Over a third of the waste in the average landfill site is paper, although this is an excellent material for recycling. Paper production consumes large quantities of energy and water, and the bleaches, dyes and other chemicals used contribute to air and water pollution (as well as posing a danger to human health when we use bleached paper – see Chapter 12, p. 186). The plantations of fast-growing conifers which provide most of our paper pulp lead to the degradation of precious countryside and the loss of important wildlife habitats. Trees play an essential and irreplaceable role in the earth's ecological systems, and their destruction is a factor contributing to the greenhouse effect.

Vera Elliott, founder of the Centre for Environmental Initiatives in Sutton, Surrey, says that no matter what subject she talks about at a meeting she is always asked what to do with newspapers. The price paid for low-quality paper by recycling buyers has made it virtually impossible for voluntary organizations to justify the time and money required to collect, sort and bundle old newspapers. Asking that your newspaper be printed on recycled paper is as important as recycling old papers.

▶ *Reduce*. Consider cutting down on the number of papers you buy. How many of us claim never to have time to read a book, but spend many hours each month reading the paper?

Save yourself aggravation and time by having your name removed from mailing lists. See Sources for the address of the Mailing Preference Service, which can have your name taken off participating companies' mailing lists. However, this won't stop everything. Why not prepare a photocopied note saying that because you are concerned about the environment and paper waste, you do not want your name sold to any other firm? Enclose a copy whenever you join an organization or subscribe to a magazine.

▶ *Reuse*. Newspapers can be used as firelighters, for making paper hats and boats, paper patterns, homemade 'peat' pots, underlay for carpeting, or as a disposable doormat. You can turn them into papier mâché.

Substantial amounts of newspaper can be turned into efficient 'logs' for your fireplace with a hand-operated machine available by mail order. This is an ideal way to make use of old papers – yours and those of the neighbours – and provides a pleasant occupation for children.

Cut attractive cards in half and use the front as a postcard next time you need to drop a note to a friend. Save sheets of paper that have been used on one side for drafting notes or for children to draw on. And of course there are many envelope labels available, which can be used to cover over the old address on the front or to reseal an envelope you have opened with a paper knife.

▶ *Buy recycled.* You can help stop the unnecessary cutting down of trees by buying products made from recycled paper. Most recycled paper requires no raw material, cuts energy consumption, and reduces air and water pollution by up to 50 per cent. It creates jobs, and saves money on waste collection and disposal.

Recycled paper used to be coarse but its quality has improved by leaps and bounds thanks to increased demand. You can now buy fine stationery, photocopying and art papers, and glossy board made from recycled paper. Choose recycled paper whenever you can. It is possible to buy loo rolls made of unbleached, recycled paper (see Sources).

Watch the labels. One fast-food chain has printed 'recyclable paper' on some of its packaging next to the international recycling symbol. That is, it is not made from recycled paper but could be recycled just like any other paper! This is the equivalent of labelling food edible.

■Recycling In The Office

▶ Send circulars rather than individual copies
▶ Use string to tie packages, rather than layers of plastic tape
▶ Reuse paper, making double-sided printing a standard practice
▶ Reuse files, ring binders and envelopes when presentation doesn't matter a great deal
▶ Reuse packing materials and boxes, or find someone who needs them
▶ Recycle newspapers, high quality office paper (which can fetch a higher price), glass and drinks cans

STRATEGIES FOR THE FUTURE

Long live the British pinta! Glass is far better reused than recycled, and this would become easier for both consumers and manufacturers if there were standard sizes for all bottles and jars.

Parts and materials from all kinds of manufactured goods can be reused or recycled into new parts. Rank Xerox is one company at the forefront of this industrial recycling, stripping old equipment down, and rebuilding new machines with restored and recycled components. Remanufacturing is an essential component in recycling strategies.

The European Union (EU) plans to require manufacturers and retailers to recover 90 per cent of packaging for recycling, and the British government is set to impose recycling costs on industry as well. In Germany, consumers have the right to return packaging and demand that it be recycled by manufacturers. Development of sympathetic packaging is slow, but as the demand for landfill sites and disposal problems grow more intense, there will be more public and legislative pressure for alternatives.

Local initiatives are growing. For example, in Wye, Kent, a community business called WyeCycle has introduced a range of recycled products and refillable containers, available only at village shops to promote local shopping. Contact your local authority to find out what they are doing now and how they plan to comply with EU directives. Recycling needs to be much easier. At the moment, conscientious recycling can takes hours a week and presents a seemingly endless stream of questions. What to save, where to take it, how to pack it – and what about the labels and the metal rings?

Recycling is going to become part of our lives and we should be preparing our homes for it now. The key is to make it easy, unobtrusive and completely routine. Once you are organized, you'll be able to cope with the vagaries of today's recycling, and ready for the more efficient schemes which are coming, and we will all adopt a more appreciative, frugal attitude towards the things which pass through our hands – seeing them as resources, not rubbish.

5

FOOD TO
SUSTAIN US

We are what we eat. Food sustains us, as a continual part of our daily lives and the source of one of life's basic pleasures. Most human cultures have made basic choices about where to live and how to organize themselves based on the availability of food, and many important rites are associated with the planting, harvesting, preparation and sharing of food.

Eating is a social act and cooking is satisfyingly creative. But in the late twentieth century food and eating have become fraught with anxiety. Food is the second largest budget item for most families, after shelter, but expense isn't the main reason for our anxiety. It may stem from the fact that we have less and less time to cook, and less and less contact with the producers of the food we eat. And we hear continually about its dangers: cholesterol, pesticides, dioxins, additives.

The green kitchen is central to *The Green Home*. The purchase, preparation and consumption of food have important ecological consequences, and problems in the environment outside have direct effects on the quality and safety of our food. Our shopping choices – the shops we choose to go to, the way our food is processed and packaged, and the individual items we buy

– have consequences, too. Fortunately, the changes that will improve your health, and make you feel more confident about the food you serve, and give your family greater pleasure in eating together, will also benefit the environment.

FOOD AND THE ENVIRONMENT

In the nineteenth century, with the use of iron tools and the availability of fossil fuels, the trend in agriculture has been to use increasingly specialized equipment, more fossil fuels and chemicals, fewer people and more land. This has especially been so since the end of the Second World War, when the possibility of producing vastly higher yields became feasible with the use of powerful chemical fertilizers. Some saw these changes as a revolution that could benefit society as a whole: more food and more leisure thanks to modern science.

The growing and transporting and processing of food is now a major international business, but agricultural policy and practice are in confusion. Famine in the third world stands in lamentable contrast to costly over-production in the first world. In the 1980s beef was being raised in Ethiopia and shipped to England, while Ethiopians starved, and the cash cropping of developing countries continues. There is a worldwide problem with soil degradation and soil erosion, and the battle against insect damage to crops is proving far more costly than anyone could have imagined when chemical pesticides first appeared. Common pesticides are affecting our health, while farm workers are exposed to more chemical hazards than most factory workers.

Nitrate fertilizers, used in vast quantities in industrial agriculture, are being washed into our lakes and streams, and turning up in our drinking water. The use of these fertilizers, and greater economic pressures, has led farmers to abandon traditional soil building methods and crop rotation in favour of intensive cultivation of only a few crops. Gains in grain production have been impressive but soil loss figures are even more staggering: in some places, more tonnes of topsoil are lost than food produced.

Nitrates from chemical fertilizers are also absorbed into plant tissue, in higher concentrations from artificial sources than from natural nitrogen-rich fertilizers like manure, and we ingest them in the food we eat. They have been associated with various forms of stomach cancer, and other health problems in children and adults.

Small farmers struggle to survive all over the world and the rural population continues to decline. Land is not cared for. Farmers are threatened with the uncertain effects of the holes in the ozone layer (with a resultant increase in ultraviolet rays) and the 'greenhouse effect' (rising CO_2 levels and global temperature, resulting from the burning of fossil fuels).

In Britain in recent years, farmers have had to cope with radiation from Chernobyl in Russia, scandals over salmonella in eggs, 'mad cow disease' (BSE) – and the pressures to use more chemicals continue.

PESTICIDES

It's estimated that since the 1940s pesticide use has increased more than tenfold while crop losses to insects have doubled. Pesticides have by no means removed the problem of dealing with pests. Even conventional growers are cutting back on chemical use with a method called integrated pest management (IPM), simply because it is a more effective way of dealing with insect pests.

In any case, killing off insects would not be to our advantage, even if we were able to do so. Insects as well as natural vegetation have an essential place in the scheme of things. Farmers depend on wild pollinators – bees and other insects – more than most of us realize. We need insects and the wild plants of meadow and hedgerow and mountainside, for practical as well as aesthetic reasons.

We are only now seeing the effects of modern pesticide use and the results of recent surveys are alarming. A leading hypothesis for the drastic decline in male fertility over the past decade, as well as for early menstruation and female sexual development, and for the growing rate of breast cancer, is that there has been an increased ingestion through food and water of the female hormone oestrogen, from sources including the use of hormones as growth promoters in cattle and pesticides which appear to mimic oestrogen. Hormonally related problems are increasing in men, too. Prostate and testicular cancer have more than doubled over past decades, and men are getting breast cancer, too.

Fungicides are thought to be particularly dangerous. They are most often used on crops from warm, humid climates, but a recent government survey found illegal or excessive levels of pesticide residues – including two fungicides classified as probable human carcinogens and another banned in Britain in 1991 – on British lettuce grown under glass. Farmers say that they cannot compete with other EU growers without fungicides to combat grey mould. The wax used to coat produce including apples, peppers, cucumbers, citrus fruits and aubergines, to improve their appearance and increase shelf life, can also contain fungicides. A detergent will remove some of this, but labels in Germany tell consumers not to use the peel from sprayed citrus fruits.

PROCESSING AND TRANSPORT

The cost of processing, storing and distributing food in the UK comes to over 50 per cent of the total food bill. While processing is not in itself a bad thing – after all, people have preserved and stored food for thousands of years – these costs are excessive and have serious environmental repercussions. Buying processed or ready-prepared food does not cut waste. The waste just goes somewhere else, with attendant energy and disposal costs.

'Fresh' fruits and vegetables are not necessarily fresh. They may have been shipped thousands of miles and kept in cold storage for months. These lengthy delays lead to deterioration of food value, especially the volatile vitamins A and C. One food scientist tested supermarket Brussels sprouts and cabbage and found no detectable vitamin C! Fruits stored for long periods need extra doses of pesticides and fungicides to preserve them, and there is a substantial energy cost involved in storage and transportation.

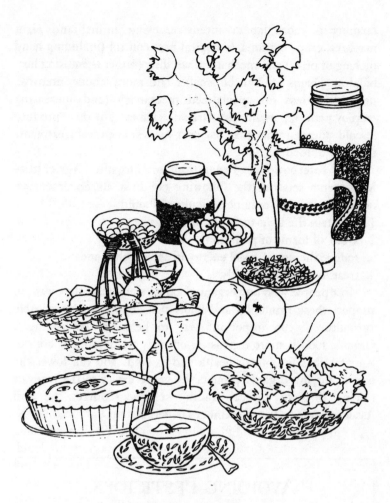

ECOLOGICAL EATING

I didn't shop for organic food until my son was six months old and I started to think about what solid food to start him on. I realized that I didn't want him to have anything which could possibly be contaminated with dangerous chemicals. His first food was scrapings of organically grown pears and our switch to organic food has progressed from there.

Organic food costs more and is thus, for the moment anyway, the provender of the better-off. The reasons are several. Organic farming is more labour intensive, using animal and plant manures, crop rotations, biological pest control (including hand picking of pests) and mechanical weeding (rather than using herbicides). Farms tend to be smaller and more labour intensive, depending less on specialized machinery (and increasing employment opportunities). Organic farmers put their produce in cold storage rather than use post-harvest chemical treatments to preserve food.

The International Federation of Organic Agriculture Movements sets out the following points in its document on organic standards: organic agriculture should:

1. maintain the long-term fertility of soils;
2. avoid all forms of pollution;
3. reduce the use of fossil energy in agriculture; and
4. treat livestock humanely.

Most people who buy organic food do so because they want to support these principles and know that supporting sustainable agriculture is an important way to help the environment. Organic food is more expensive, but it is an investment both in your family's long-term health and in land. You can lower the cost of buying organic produce by going direct to the farm or buying through a local trading scheme (contact the Soil Association for a list of member farmers).

AVOIDING PESTICIDES

- Start an organic garden (see Chapter 15).
- Whenever you can, buy organic.
- Press for comprehensive labelling of fresh fruits and vegetables.
- Beware of perfect-looking produce. Many chemical pesticides are used to enhance the appearance of the food. A few superficial flaws do not affect the quality or flavour of what you buy.

- Wash all produce which has not been grown organically. Plain water or a mild solution of biodegradable washing up liquid and water will remove some, but not all, of the surface pesticide residues.
- Peel produce when appropriate. This means extra work and losing some of the valuable nutrients contained in fresh food, but will completely remove surface residues.
- Buy domestically grown produce in season – these generally contain fewer pesticide residues (many cookbooks have guides to when fruits and vegetables are in season, and therefore cheapest).

■Local Food

While at least a little home-grown food is within everyone's reach (if only sprouted lentils and a few windowbox herbs), most of us depend on whatever shops offer. The Safe Alliance, an umbrella group of British farmers, environmentalists, third world and animal welfare activists, is campaigning to make people aware of the way imported fruits and vegetables have pushed home grown food off the shelves. Supermarkets import food from Chile, Tasmania, Israel and Kenya. This is not a matter of buying special produce that does not grow in Britain. We buy apples from France and carrots from California, and British farmers are suffering as a result.

The Safe Alliance has suggested that the government change its Food From Britain promotion agency to a domestic promotion aimed at encouraging people to buy home grown food. The only people gaining from this trade are transport and oil companies, and international agribusiness and chemical companies. The consumer is getting food which is less fresh and less nutritious, and the prices do not reflect the true costs to people and the environment of producing and transporting food around the world. At present about 70 per cent of the organic food sold in the UK comes from abroad because there are insufficient domestic supplies to meet demand.

One serious danger with food from the third world is that agricultural chemicals which are banned in the West are exported to third world countries, so we can be consuming trace chemicals which have been proved to be cancer-causing or mutagenic. Recent trials in the US have found that pesticide residues on imported fruits and vegetables were higher than on domestic produce, and the types of pesticides were often more hazardous.

Thinking about using local produce has changed the way I shop. While it is pleasant to be able to buy French cider, Italian parmesan and Greek olives, this may lead us to ignore and undervalue Devon cider, Welsh butter, Stilton cheese and innumerable other British specialities, and the products of your own region. Try to find local sources for some of your food. A neighbour may be willing to sell their excess from a flourishing garden; there may be farms nearby where you can buy eggs or milk or honey; and there are city farms in urban areas.

WHAT ABOUT MEAT?

Vegetarians and vegans have substantially lower rates of heart disease and cancer, lower blood pressure and cholesterol levels, and tend to be slimmer than meat eaters. Although in the third world many people don't get enough protein, we get more than enough without meat or soya bean substitutes. Premature ageing and degenerative diseases have been associated with eating too much protein.

Butchers feel beleaguered, what with all the publicity about the evils of animal fats and intensive farming practices. Public awareness about dietary fibre has made many of us shift to eating more pulses and whole grains and less meat. To make matters worse, my local butcher tells me that people just aren't willing to pay high prices for a good piece of beef.

There is no way to identify a chicken contaminated with salmonella and a *Which?* test found that three out of five British chickens are contaminated with food poisoning bacteria. Reported food poisoning cases continue to rise, with 69,000 examples in 1993. Infection has spread rapidly because of intensive rearing and modern slaughtering methods, designed to produce cheap food for a large market. Battery-reared chickens and other animals are kept under barbaric conditions, and the ecological impact of factory farming is profound.

In addition, the waste involved in commercial meat production is taking food out of the mouths of starving people when the grain fed to animals comes from the third world. More than half the world's grain harvest goes to feed livestock, an enormous and inexcusable waste of food that could feed human beings.

In the light of these points, most environmentalists promote what is called 'eating low on the food chain'. To produce 1lb of beef requires 16lb of grain, as well as considerable inputs of water; this concentration of protein is expensive, inefficient and also concentrates pesticides found in the grain or other feed. Pork is more efficient, requiring 6lb of feed to produce 1lb of meat, and the rate for chickens and eggs is about three to one.

Traditional cuisines in most parts of the world – including Europe – have used meat primarily as a seasoning or special treat, and many cuisines becoming more popular in Britain use little or no meat. Eating from a wider variety of cuisines has helped to break the 'meat and two veg' routine for many of us (though female friends complain that it is hard to persuade their men of this, and I struggle with my husband and children over their passion for meat and potatoes).

Veganism means eating no animal products whatsoever, with the possible exception of honey. In our society this is a demanding choice, especially because you eliminate those great instant foods, eggs and cheese. Substitutes are often made of soyabeans and take considerable processing. You might want to consult a vegan cookbook for occasional ideas. Most wholefood and vegetarian restaurants now provide vegan dishes. Vegans also use synthetic materials to replace leather and wool, something of a problem in environmental terms.

■Responsible Meat Eating

There is much to be said for the rearing of animals as part of a sustainable agriculture. Virtually all cultures throughout history have used animals for food, in the form of milk, blood and meat, and traditional farming methods depend on animal manures. 'Mixed farming' creates a neat ecological cycle: animals graze fallow land and eat scraps which would otherwise be wasted (free-range chickens do even more: they eat large numbers of pests), and provide manure to fertilize the next crop.

For those who are content to eat little or no meat much of the time but who do not want to give it up entirely, there is now a 'real meat' movement, making it possible to eat meat from animals raised without routine antibiotics, growth promoters and hormones, without chemical additives or water being added to the meat. A number of butchers sell real meat and you can order by post. Talk to your butcher about stocking it (promise to buy the meat yourself and to tell all your friends).

Other suppliers sell meat from rare breeds, which means that you can promote biodiversity while you grill your pork chops. These old-fashioned meats, from Southdown sheep and Gloucester Old Spot pigs, are more expensive than intensively reared meat but they have a robust flavour so you can get away with serving less.

If you are buying from the supermarket, lamb is probably a better bet than other commercially reared meat because sheep are primarily range animals, not stock fed with grain. Sheep and goats are crucial in many societies, producing milk, meat and leather for clothing from land which is unsuitable for farming. Stick to free-range chicken, game and fish as much as possible. While offal is nutritious – and delicious – these organs, especially the liver, tend to store poisons. Avoid them if you do not have a source of organic meat.

ENDANGERED SPECIES

One of the problems with modern agriculture is the tiny range of any individual crop grown commercially, by chemical or organic methods. There are thousands of varieties of any given fruit or vegetable, as you will know if you look through a seed catalogue (and seed catalogues by no means have all possible varieties – see 'Seed Savers', Chapter 15, p. 246). But the potatoes, cauliflowers and strawberries we buy come from an extremely limited range of varieties; the 'popular' varieties are the ones growers like: they look good, have bigger yields and grow larger, travel well and can stand storage. Eating quality or taste is not a commercial criterion. Foodies insist we need to go back to old vegetable varieties and breed again, this time concentrating on flavour, diversity, local adaptation and adaptability in the kitchen.

Even our grains are limited. We eat wheat, mostly Canadian, and maize, a native American crop, and rice, an Asian one. The wheat and oats grown in Britain today are more suited to arid Turkish hillsides than to our rainy island climate, while we eat little of the oats, barley and rye our ancestors grew.

PROMOTING BIODIVERSITY

- Grow your own food or buy locally grown food.
- Choose local and old varieties when you see them: Slack-My-Girdle and Ellison's Orange apples, for example. Attend an apple tasting or pick apples from an old orchard.
- Eat the unusual: try blue corn instead of yellow, small plantains instead of large bananas (though of course these are not local crops).
- Serve traditional drinks: scrumpy, perry, country wines.
- Buy a variety of fruits and vegetables, including some of the new potatoes available.
- Eat seasonally: use cabbage instead of hothouse, fungicide-sprayed lettuce for winter salads, and enjoy strawberries and new potatoes in spring.
- Buy white eggs if brown are common, to encourage farms to raise more than one species of chicken (colour is determined by species, not by rearing method).
- Order meat from one of the farmers who raises rare old breeds.

HEALTHY EATING

Most of us know the basics for healthy eating: less fat and sugar, more fresh fruits and vegetables, less meat and more roughage. The most important thing to remember, if you want to improve your eating habits, is 'Good food I like'. This is a lot more constructive than concentrating on the bad things you eat and feel guilty about.

Concentrate on good food before considering nutritional supplements. There are a number of nutritious foods which you can emphasize in your diet – seaweeds, yoghurt, garlic, brewer's yeast – which are wholefoods, not health foods. How do you rate a natural foods store? Look for a large selection of simply packaged whole grains, legumes, nuts and dried fruits; a reasonable range of organically grown produce in good condition; and cool cabinets with untreated milk, yoghurt and cheese, tofu and tempeh products.

GOOD FATS

One of the major health debates of the past two decades has been over the role of fats in our diet. Margarine is one of the most highly refined foods in the modern diet, yet health-conscious people have eaten it because of worries about cholesterol. The public has now been thoroughly indoctrinated with the idea that saturated fats are bad, though there is considerable disagreement among scientists about the role of cholesterol in heart disease and much recent evidence that a diet high in polyunsaturated oils is bad for your health. There has never been conclusive evidence that lowering blood cholesterol saves lives, nor of a clear relationship between diet and cholesterol levels.

Everyone seems to argue that monosaturated olive oil is good for us, though the exact reasons remain unclear. One of the good things about extra virgin olive oil is that it is pressed, not extracted with solvents from plant material like other vegetable oils. Commercial vegetable oils are a recent development. They are extracted with petrochemical solvents such as benzene or methylene chloride, known carcinogens, and are then bleached and deodorized. The late Jane Grigson, author of a number of excellent cookery books, wrote that she preferred to stick to natural butter, lard, and olive oil. I'm with her: I cannot believe that a highly refined product containing traces of hazardous chemicals is better for me than natural, unrefined foods.

Too much unsaturated fat seems to depress the immune system and promote tumour growth; some researchers suspect that the increased use of polyunsaturate fats has contributed to the high incidence of cancer in Western civilization. Unsaturated fats – containing essential fatty acids – are indeed needed for good health, but only in small amounts. They should come from a natural, untreated source such as fresh raw seeds, unrefined oils or fish and fish oils. Biscuits and cakes in which vegetable fats are listed as an ingredient are likely to contain highly saturated palm or coconut oils, or hydrogenated vegetable oils.

▶ Reduce fats from all sources. Good fats recommended below are more expensive than those you've probably been using, an excellent deterrent to over-consumption.

▶ Use unrefined, mechanically pressed (sometimes called first pressing or extra virgin) oil and heat them as little as possible. They should be stored in a cool place.

▶ Cold-pressed oils have distinctive flavours, unlike bland commercial oils. You'll need to experiment to find ones you like. Sunflower and safflower oils are quite strong; corn oil is milder. Sesame oil (not the dark, toasted kind used as a flavouring) is also bland. On salads, use olive oil, or delicious walnut or hazelnut oil.

▶ Buy organically grown oils and butter from organic herds. Pesticides and other chemicals concentrate in fats, both animal and vegetable.

▶ If you deep fry, use fresh oil each time. Heating alters the chemical structure of oils.

▶ Use butter (in small amounts) in preference to highly processed margarine.

▶ Choose organic dairy products whenever you can, and buy

meat which has been produced without antibiotics, growth promoters and hormones.

▶ Cut the fat off your meat and choose lean cuts, especially at the supermarket. Fatty meat will contain higher levels of pesticide residues than lean meat.

▶ Lard is a useful cooking fat, but commercial varieties contain traces of pesticides and growth promoters, and also have added antioxidants as preservatives. To get traditional lard you will almost certainly have to make your own.

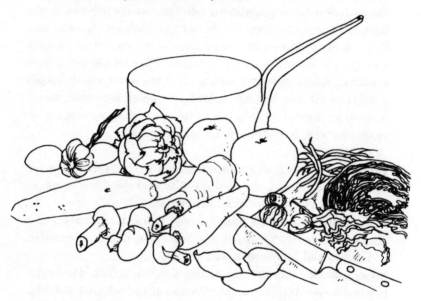

THE ECOLOGICAL KITCHEN

Ecological eating is nothing new. The native cuisines of cultures around the world have developed in modest family kitchens, where meals were produced from the least expensive and most abundant local foods.

Having the right equipment and a range of basic ingredients and seasonings is essential to producing meals with ease. Favourite recipes should be in an accessible spot; it's a good idea to keep cookbooks in or near the kitchen, rather than above your desk or in the bedroom. You need their inspiration and information near at hand.

It's important to be creative about the way we eat. Sometimes it seems that prepackaged and takeaway meals are the only way to cope with hectic modern schedules, but that isn't quite true. Many people with busy lives and little time manage to eat proper, albeit simple, meals.

Ensure that you always have a supply of things you don't need to cook: fruit, vegetable sticks, yoghurt, cheese and good bread. Even small children can make an adequate supper on these. Make out a list of your own rock bottom six easy meals, just to prove that you can get through a week of eating at home: baked potatoes, omelettes or scrambled eggs, pasta, grilled fish, cheese and salad, stir-fried vegetables, for example. That'll take you through a week, at a pinch. The seventh night you eat at your mother's, cadge a meal from a friend who loves to cook or go to a restaurant.

See Chapter 7 for suggestions about saving energy in the kitchen. A simple way is to allow dishes to cook in their own heat. Nutritionist Adelle Davis recommended bringing a soup or spaghetti sauce to a boil, turning off the flame and allowing the pan to stand rather than simmer for a couple of hours – boil the sauce thoroughly afterwards, to kill any bacteria.

You can save yourself work and save energy by doubling or even tripling recipes. It's not much more trouble to make a huge batch of lasagne than a tiny one. Eat some now, and chill or freeze the rest for another meal. If possible, freeze food in a dish it can be reheated in; a collection of cheap glass baking dishes makes this easy. Be careful, however, if you're an inexperienced cook: cakes don't always take to doubling – check your big basic cookbook for guidance.

HOME COOKING SIMPLIFIED

- Stock your pantry with staples that last.
- Buy in bulk so you never run out of crucial ingredients.
- Buy simple foods you really enjoy.
- Get a wide range of pots and pans (see below).
- Make the small touches grand, and keep the big things simple. Serve local smoked trout as a starter, then serve an easy pasta dish as a main course.
- Cook in pans that leftover food can be stored in.
- Store food in pans that can go into the oven.
- Install a dishwasher. Avoid using the drying cycle, opening the machine instead to let dishes dry naturally.
- Eat with the children. Experts say a light, early supper is better for health and your waistline. But eat after the children have gone to bed at least once a week, to remind yourself of what civilized dining at home is all about.

■Pots And Pans

The best pans are expensive but they last for ever and encourage home cooking. There are a few health issues to keep in mind as you choose cookware. Metals are soluble: even stainless steel (made of steel, chromium and nickel) needs to be looked after with care. Trace amounts of nickel, a toxic metal, are found in acidic foods cooked in stainless steel – not enough to bother most of us, but some health experts advise against refrigerating food in a stainless steel pan.

A far greater concern is aluminium, which has been associated with a number of brain disorders. Aluminium, too, dissolves in acidic foods. Have you noticed how an aluminium pan sparkles if you cook rhubarb or apple sauce in it? Tea is acid, so throw out aluminium teapots.

If Teflon-coated pans are put over a high flame they release toxic fumes. Enamelled pans, such as Le Creuset, are excellent.

Glass is inert so it's a good choice if you worry about metal contamination, but it doesn't conduct heat well.

Studies show that food cooked in iron pans have twice the iron of foods cooked in glass or enamel, and the iron is as available to the body as the iron in beef. If you are iron deficient, cooking in cast iron could improve your diet. It's also cheap and durable, and conducts heat better than anything else.

AVOIDING WASTE

Even though clearing our plates is not going to save a child in the Sudan from starvation, a more conscious and appreciative attitude towards the food we buy will reduce waste and save some money – money that might actually help a starving child.

A rare culinary skill these days is making full use of every bit of food. Of course most of us don't have farmhouse kitchens or time to make our own sausages, but we could make far better use of the food we buy. To make good use of food and avoid waste, someone has to pay attention to the shopping and the pantry shelves, and it takes a bit of time.

▶ Budget cookbooks are full of ideas for making the most of what you buy.

▶ Leftovers may have become something of a joke but in fact many foods taste better the second day. Establish one area of the fridge for things to be used up so the family will look there for a piece of lasagne to warm for lunch. I also have a system for storing dregs of wine for cooking, stock ingredients like the juice from a tin of tomatoes and paper butter wrappers for greasing tins.

▶ It's more important to find a use for good Cheddar that's starting to dry up at the edges than for the odd crust of bread. Make the most of expensive ingredients.

▶ Simplify, simplify. Why peel potatoes? It's been estimated that each year the average family throws away in its potato peelings the amount of vitamin C in 95 glasses of orange juice, the iron in 500 eggs and the protein in 60 steaks. Scrub them with a good brush, cut out eyes and spots – without worrying about the occasional blemish – and make them into mashed potatoes, or home fries or chips, exactly as they are.

▶ Soup is the ideal vehicle for oddments. Making a classic clear meat stock is complicated but one can make delicious broth, to eat as it is or use as a soup base, with casual techniques from food that would otherwise be wasted. Decent meaty bones should be browned in a little fat (or use a turkey carcass, or even bones snagged from family plates if you're not fussy) before you add water and some vegetables for flavouring, perhaps onions, carrots and celery, bay leaf and parsley. Salt will draw out the flavours and I often add dregs of wine or a dash of vinegar to extract calcium from the bones.

▶ Candying citrus peel is easy, it makes a lovely gift, and makes the price of organically grown oranges and grapefruits much easier to justify (see the instructions in Jane Grigson's *Fruit Book*).

FAST FOOD

An increasing number of British meals are eaten out of the home. In environmental terms, this is a mixed blessing. Restaurant eating can be a good thing, as restaurants purchase foods in bulk (saving packaging) and preparing them in large quantities (saving energy). But many restaurants, even expensive ones, serve pre-packaged and processed foods. Good ethnic restaurants may be the best choice, and you can always ask if the vegetables are fresh or frozen when you order, and whether the soup is home made.

Fast food restaurants have been maligned by environmentalists, food and labour activists for their contribution to the destruction of tropical rainforests and loss of biological diversity (see Chapter 3, p. 39), for their unfair treatment of employees, for the huge amounts of plastic and paper waste they add to the 'disposal stream' and litter to our streets, and because they give us proverbially unhealthy food.

One of the problems with having commercially prepared meals available at all hours is that we've forgotten the pleasures of the simple meals our ancestors enjoyed after a day's work: good bread, cheese, a glass of beer. Lay in a supply of wholesome, non-perishable and almost instantaneous food. Try to avoid tinned foods but a few tins – good soups and beans and tuna – make a good addition to the impromptu meal shelf.

People in every urban area eat fast food, but traditional street food was sold by individuals as a way to earn a living, and it made use of local, seasonal ingredients and had real character. In ecological terms, buying a takeaway from a locally owned restaurant is better than buying one from a hamburger chain.

FOOD ON THE GO

Not only is the food at motorway stops and on most trains heavily processed and wrapped, for the most part it is pretty awful to eat. You can enjoy better food and save money by ensuring that you always have basic picnic equipment in the glovebox or your overnight case. During the day you can stop at a market or shop to buy provisions – and if you travel with one of the food guides listed in Sources you can often pick up a regional speciality along the way.

It is possible to assemble a pleasant and satisfying meal if you have the following supplies with you: a sharp knife; corkscrew; a few pieces of cutlery; small hand towels to use as napkins and for wiping up; salt and pepper, mustard, vinegar. Carry real mugs along to avoid getting takeaway coffee or tea in a plastic cup (saves waste and tastes much better). With an old-fashioned wicker picnic basket you can transport wine glasses, and a tiny camping stove makes it possible to brew a fresh cuppa.

For long journeys pack a basket with a plentiful supply of drinks and snack foods. A big flask of iced water is good in warm weather and in the winter there is nothing more welcome than hot apple juice spiked with cinnamon. Bottles or cartons of juice, crackers, cheese, fresh fruit, raw vegetables, and dried fruit and nuts travel well, and are easy to eat.

SLOW FOOD

While market research shows that more people are grazing – grabbing meals on the run, heating ready-prepared food in the microwave – some of us are trying to buck the trend. Certainly the demand for large kitchens is a good sign; more family members can contribute to food preparation, and cooking becomes a shared event, a chance to reconnect with one another. The market for cookery books and classes shows that there are many people who understand that food is not simply fuel and that eating good food is one of the great pleasures of life.

In 1986, Italian journalist Carlo Petrini founded an organization and publishing company dedicated to Slow Food, aiming to promote a pace of life at which mealtimes can be valued as a time of conviviality and gastronomic pleasure. The organization, Arcigola Slow Food in Cuneo, Italy, supports traditional family-run restaurants with its popular guidebook *Osterie d'Italia*, and is credited with saving some of these *osterias* from extinction.

Of course it isn't always easy to make time for real meals together. But like other suggestions in *The Green Home*, a switch from fast food to slow food is not all or nothing, nor is it something that happens all at once. Slow food can be very simple: hot pancakes fresh off the griddle and eaten dripping with syrup or smoky-hot jacket potatoes with country cheese. Busy Americans like casual 'potluck' parties where everyone contributes one course. Eating together is an important human experience, which makes your world a better place. Give yourself time to enjoy it. *Bon appetit!*

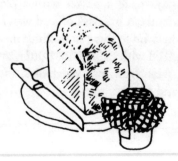

6

WHERE WE LIVE –LAND AND SHELTER

Our homes come from the earth: they are built of stone or straw, brick or reed, wood or clay. Most people throughout history have made their homes out of the materials at hand, whether carved into hills of compacted volcanic ash in Turkey or built of flint and thatch from the Sussex marshes. A human dwelling – however it is shaped and whatever it is made of – is the most enduring, and expensive, investment we make.

Dwellings have great significance in our lives. Shelter is their primary and essential function, but home is not merely a roof over our heads. Our homes are where we retire for rest, and sustenance and safety, where major events of loving and grieving and rejoicing take place. Our homes are the theatres of our lives, the places we share with the people dearest to us.

'Home' is also more than the buildings we live in. Our sense of home depends on external features, in the garden or down the street, that make up our area or village or parish or city.

While *The Green Home* is primarily about the way we live in our homes, in this chapter we look at where we live and aspects of livability that go beyond our four walls. The way we as a society live shapes the homes we live in, and the way our neighbourhoods and towns are designed. The rapid changes in transport and work patterns of the past few decades have had a devastating impact on community life. And aspects of the environment around us affect our health and well-being, for good or ill. Many people have become involved in environmental campaigns as a result of a particular issue threatening their own area.

THE BRITISH LANDSCAPE

The British countryside is, in part, a human artefact and includes some of the most ancient farm landscapes in Europe. We humans have been altering the landscape for thousands of years, so in one sense modern changes are nothing new. What is new is the pace, scope and size of the changes. The earth is very accommodating. Plants and animals move to new locations as old ones grow infertile or inhospitable, but they generally do this over many generations. Today, acres can be cleared in a day. When I look at children's books about the destruction of the rainforests, a picture forms in my mind of bulldozers widening the M25.

The impact of roads has in itself forever altered the British landscape, both visually and biologically. The landscapes we know are the result of intricate interactions of climate, soil, landforms, plants and animals, forming what biologists call ecosystems. A sheet of hard exposed surface, continually travelled by high speed metal objects, poses an insurmountable barrier to many animals. Noise drives them away, and toxic fumes pollute their food and water. Roads are considered a major threat to biodiversity, breaking up ecological systems in such a way that many species are lost, and they are changing the character of the towns and villages that are an essential part of much of the British landscape.

TREES

Trees, too, are vital to our sense of place. Trees make special and memorable spots, where people meet and muse. A mighty oak or ash, or an orchard of apple and pear trees, is one of the beauties of town or countryside, and trees perform vital functions, improving air quality, creating habitats for birds and insects, and cooling streets and buildings.

In spite of our vaunted love of trees and our concern about the trees of the rainforests, England today has only 7 per cent tree cover. In the EU, only Ireland has fewer trees, and the Countryside Commission has urged the government to make all effort to increase the amount of land set aside for tree planting.

Existing trees are under threat. Cable television is creating a new environmental problem, as more than a hundred cable franchises licensed by the Department of Trade and Industry lay cables along an estimated 50 miles of streets each day. Pavements are dug up, cables laid and the trenches covered over. The damage is not immediately visible: tree roots may have been severed or damaged, and thousands of trees are dying a lingering death.

Trees have a tough time surviving in city streets even without the threat of root damage. They suffer from drought and pollution, and have often been planted without proper soil preparation. Planting trees is one of the best things we can do for the environment as a whole, but it needs to be done thoughtfully. Get advice from a gardening book, your local garden centre and write to Common Ground for information about the importance of trees.

WHERE WE LIVE

While we may long for the rural idyll, more and more of us live in cities. By the year 2010, according to the United National publication *World Organisation Prospects*, an estimated 52.8 per cent of the world's population will live in cities. Cities are becoming more crowded, polluted and unsafe, but they have had eminent proponents. Lewis Mumford, author of the epic *The City in History*, and Jane Jacobs, author of *Cities and the Wealth of Nations*, have relished the exuberance and complexity of urban life. They have many successors who are working hard to green the cities of the twenty-first century.

■The Rural Dilemma

And rural life is not always so idyllic. Local economies are failing and one rural household in five is living below the poverty line. House prices are high in rural areas: in places desirable to second home owners as much as 50 per cent above the national average. Young people are not able to live in the villages where they grew up because there are no jobs and they cannot afford a house. And the loss of services has changed the character of rural life for people on low incomes, especially for those without cars. Figures show that almost 40 per cent of parishes have no shop, 60 per cent have no primary school and 75 per cent have no general practitioner.

Threatened reductions to the train network (after the staggering cuts over the past decades) leave rural people increasingly dependent on expensive and polluting cars, while at the same time suffering the blight of new roads and increased pollution.

While tourism is an important source of income for many rural areas, tourism can contribute to the degradation of the beautiful rural Britain people come to enjoy, and tends to weaken local community ties and associations. Environment-friendly policies would concentrate on revitalizing local economies and would require developments to be planned to minimize the need to travel, by, for example, putting houses near shops, schools and services.

THINGS TO LOOK FOR IF YOU PLAN TO MOVE HOUSE

- Local schools, shops, parks and other facilities.
- Diversified public transport (buses, trains, foot and cycle paths).
- Progressive environmental policies and services (see Sources for the model environmental services charter drawn up by the Department of the Environment).
- Active citizens' groups.

■ The Legacy Of Pollution

One of the challenges facing local and national governments is land contaminated by industrial or military use. When the Environmental Protection Act was passed in 1989/90, the government intended to establish a register of contaminated land in the UK, but landowners and developers forced this plan to be abandoned. The government does not know how much of the country is contaminated – estimates range from 1000 to 2000 hectares – and some environmental groups would place the figure considerably higher. Priorities (for people who care) include the identification of contaminated land and the establishment of a clean-up system with defined liability, and priorities for dealing with the most polluted sites first.

The importance of this is considerable because it not only pushes the government to deal with past pollution but encourages industry not to pollute in future. The environmental price-tags have to include the real costs of doing business, which include clean-up costs – the polluter ought to pay for the damage caused.

The environmental problems that face us where we live are the same in urban and rural environments: traffic and industry, incineration and waste sites, pesticide spraying and radon. Our homes can shelter us only partially from these hazards, and one of the results of a greater awareness of the dangers of environmental pollution is the emergence of citizens' groups protesting about pollution or development in their area.

This has been dubbed NIMBY – Not In My Backyard – and has acquired a bad reputation for obstructiveness and selfishness. After all, the toxic waste and new housing has to go somewhere. But the people who suffer most from pollution are rarely those who create or benefit from it. NIMBYism can teach us that our consumer choices create pollution and waste we don't want to see in our areas, and that we should therefore demand products made with materials and processes that do not pollute other people's neighbourhoods or pristine wild places.

■Local Distinctiveness

One of the best-known green slogans is 'Think globally and act locally'. It makes sense to think globally in a world where rapid transportation and telecommunications have brought the world to our shops and television screens, but thinking globally can impoverish our sense of home. Thinking globally puts our attention elsewhere. Acting locally to solve global environmental problems is certainly part of what *The Green Home* is about, but we should also act locally to solve local problems.

We also need to shift our focus, now and then, away from problems and issues to the intimate realities of our connection with the environment we live in. That sense of connection depends on all the things that make one place different from another, rather than on the shop fronts and blocks of flats that look the same in Inverness and Itchen Abbas.

The arts and environmental organization Common Ground campaigns for local distinctiveness, encouraging people to make parish maps showing the natural and human-made things that make their place unique, to conserve old buildings, hedgerows, orchards, family businesses and winding lanes, to use local stone, brick and wood in new buildings, and to consider the invisible aspects of our surroundings: local dialects, archaeological remains, family histories, stories inherent in the names of fields, streets and villages.

Their slogans for the green consumer are 'resist the things that can be found anywhere' and 'demand the best of the new'. You can add features of local distinctiveness to your home by using local materials, serving local foods and drinks, decorating with old maps and prints of your area, and encouraging the diversity of local landmarks around your home. Don't tidy up too much – let old things weather gracefully.

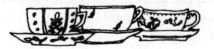

HOW WELL DO YOU KNOW THE PLACE YOU LIVE?

1. Where does your water come from? Where did it fall as precipitation, where is it treated and stored?
2. What phase is the moon in? When will the moon be full?
3. What type of soil do you live on?
4. What was the total rainfall in your area last year?
5. How long ago was your region first inhabited? Who lived there?
6. Can you name five native edible plants and the seasons when they are available?
7. From what direction do storms/winds usually come?
8. Where does your rubbish go?
9. How long is the growing season?
10. Can you name five resident and five migratory birds in your area?
11. What is the land use history of where you live?
12. What visible evidence is there in your area of geological changes that shaped the land forms you know?
13. What species have become extinct?
14. Can you point north from where you are sitting?
15. What spring wildflower blooms first where you live? When does it bloom?

(adapted from *Home! A Bioregional Reader*)

ECOLOGICAL DESIGN

Green building means more than energy-efficient windows and sustainably harvested wood doors. There is a growing movement among architects, landscape architects and industrial designers to consider the ecological implications of the buildings, parks and products they help to create.

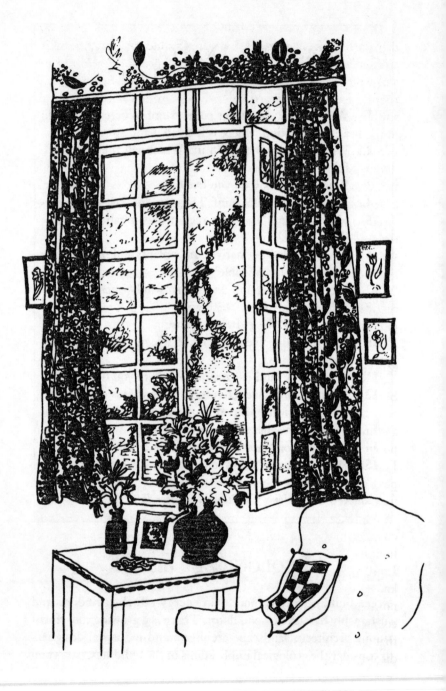

Green design includes planning ways to save trees and avoid damage to tree roots, preserve streams, reduce pollution from the construction process, and replant native species of trees, shrubs and wildflowers. Wetlands can be protected from sediment and runoff, and buildings can be designed around natural features and views. The height of buildings can be planned to keep within the height of trees.

Ecological design also includes an emphasis on vernacular design – that is, using the materials, colours, shapes and structures traditional or native to the area rather than trying to imitate a Tuscan farmhouse in the fens of Cambridgeshire. Vernacular interior design makes sense. The cosy, rather cluttered effect of the traditional British indoors, replete with bright chintzes and wood surfaces, is just right in a damp, cool climate.

If you plan to use an architect, contact the Ecological Design Association (EDA) for a referral, and if you are designing and renovating yourself, you might want to subscribe to the EDA journal *EcoDesign*.

■Timber Treatments

Serious health damage has been attributed to chemicals used for common timber treatments required by most building societies and indemnity insurers (who are only just beginning to consider potential liability for homeowners affected by toxic chemicals). Lawsuits have been brought against timber treatment firms by people whose homes were treated and former employees who now suffer from acute health problems.

While firms and government bodies are researching non-chemical ways of treating wood, products currently in use include lindane, TBTO and various pentachlorophenates. Lindane is a broad spectrum organochloride insecticide and a known carcinogen. TBTO is an extremely dangerous chemical, now banned as an antifoulant for boats and banned in many other countries for home wood treatment (German research suggests that it causes psychosis, anxiety and other central nervous system disorders).

Research into alternatives is being undertaken by the Building

Research Establishment, the Timber Research and Development Association, the National Trust and a number of universities. Permethrin is a less toxic alternative, developed for use in buildings where bats live. It is an analogue of pyrethrum, a natural, plant-based insecticide used by organic gardeners, and has become popular because people think it may also be less toxic for humans. Another alternative is inorganic boron.

Heat treatment can be used to treat woodworm in small pieces of furniture and in Denmark it is used to kill dry rot. Some commercial timber treatment firms will, if requested, use non-chemical methods to treat fungal decay: by cutting out all rotten timber, removing sources of damp and then carefully monitoring moisture levels. This sort of treatment is more expensive than chemical treatment, and does not come with the thirty-year guarantees that almost all building societies require (the Ecology Building Society is the single exception).

As in human health care, prevention is the best remedy. Careful design and maintenance can eliminate the need for rot treatment, and the use of suitable hardwoods could minimize problems too (the cheaper, unseasoned woods used today are more vulnerable to rot).

If you are buying a new home, contact the London Hazards Centre or the Ecological Design Association for further information.

■Building Materials

Good materials are biodegradable, low in energy consumption and not based on depletable resources, and making them should not pollute the environment. In Germany there are 'biological' architects, and firms which supply ecologically sound and non-toxic building and decorating materials, and in Britain the EDA is now promoting the wider use of green building materials and methods.

In the mean time, when you start building or decorating, look for natural, unprocessed materials. This means wallpaper made of paper rather than plastic, wood, cork or tile floors, and wool carpets or cotton rugs. Many people choose these things because they are inherently more pleasant to live with and because they usually last longer than synthetics. And when they do wear out, they won't be lingering in a landfill site for hundreds of years.

New homes are likely to have large amounts of plastic and pressed woods (bound with urea-formaldehyde resin) which it would be both difficult and expensive to replace. This is another incentive for using old furniture and fittings, and improving old housing stock whenever possible. If you are restoring an older home, what could be more appropriate than to use original materials, which are almost all biodegradable and non-toxic? There are many sources of both second-hand 'salvage' and good reproductions, virtually all of which will be in natural materials and designed to last.

PREFERRED MATERIALS

- **Insulation**: cellulose, perlite, vermiculite, fibreglass, rock wool, cork.
- **Weatherstripping**: metal.
- **Interior walls and ceilings**: gypsum board or plaster.
- **Caulking**: linseed oil putty, clear silicone.
- **Flooring**: brick, slate, untreated wood, concrete, ceramic tile, natural linoleum, untreated natural fibre carpets.
- **Cabinetry**: solid sustainably-harvested wood, enamelled metal.
- **Worktops**: ceramic tile, wood, granite, marble.
- **Plumbing**: copper pipes with lead-free solder or mechanical joints.

■ Good Wood

Wood is a satisfying material to work and live with, but the choices we make when we buy wood have huge environmental consequences. Britain has been importing over a million doors from tropical countries each year. These are sold through a variety of retail outlets and you may well have bought one without having the slightest idea that this is a contributing factor to the destruction of the earth's precious rainforests.

In 1988 the National Association of Retail Furnishers produced a *Good Wood Guide* to promote the use of sustainably produced timber, most of it from Europe and North America, as well as from a few well-managed tropical forests. Now major British retailers – notably B&Q – are revamping their timber buying in cooperation with the WorldWide Fund for Nature UK (WWF UK), a partnership which aims to phase out the sale and use of all unsustainable wood and wood products. B&Q explicitly concerns itself with 'underlying issues in the tropics, such as inappropriate land use and the need for development to fight poverty and debt'. WWF UK is also promoting an independent timber labelling system under the auspices of the Forest Stewardship Council.

Ask about the woods you buy. Salad bowls, wooden spoons, skirting boards and shelving should all be made from sustainably harvested and preferably native British woods. In general, tropical hardwoods such as iroko and mahogany should be avoided; even if they are sustainably harvested, there are high energy costs involved in transporting wood around the world.

■Fabrics And Furnishings

Environmental toxins come from furniture, floor coverings and other domestic fittings. People who are chemically sensitive have extreme reactions – burning feeling in lungs, rashes and headaches – and there have been many cases of so-called Sick Building Syndrome after the installation of new carpets, which are treated with a range of chemicals to make them stain-resistant, moth repellent, and to make cheap carpets look and feel more luxurious.

The resins used to bind plywood and chipboard, and to treat furnishing fabrics are significant sources of formaldehyde vapour, which is highly irritating to some people and may cause allergic reactions in children. Formaldehyde is particularly hazardous because it seems to act as a trigger for acute chemical sensitivity. After exposure to high levels of formaldehyde (after the installation of new particle board cupboards, for example) quite a number of people have become chemical cripples – unable to tolerate even small quantities of the many other human-made chemicals which surround us. Studies have found that the concentration of formaldehyde vapour in the air tripled after chipboard furniture was installed in an otherwise empty house.

Buying natural fibres may not solve the problem. Even cotton can be loaded with dyes, pesticide residues from growing and chemical residues from processing, and 'no-iron' fabrics are treated with formaldehyde resin. One of the growing trends in the bed and bath retail market is unbleached, undyed and untreated cotton sheets and towels. These creamy coloured items are softer and more comfortable, as well as better for the environment. An industry representative says that although 'natural' cotton is more expensive because it requires special handling and equipment, once production is done on a larger scale manufacturers will save money on dyes, making untreated cotton less expensive.

In addition, cotton breeders are starting to see a market for other colours of natural cotton – soft browns and greens that develop on the plant – and there are now organic cotton growers who use integrated pest management (IPM) to control insects, rather than dangerous chemical pesticides.

There are some simple solutions. Your nose is a good guide to some chemical air pollution. If a new shower curtain has a distinctive plastic smell, it is outgassing chemicals. The odour of a new rug or carpet can be removed by steam cleaning with plain water after installation. Certain smells disappear quickly and you can speed the outgassing process by improving ventilation. Have new carpets fitted in the summer when you can leave windows open, choose solid wood furniture and don't replace old chipboard if possible.

■Paints And Finishes

One of the things prospective parents always do is paint the nursery – to make it bright and pristine. They don't realize that paint can pollute the air. This is why the odour of new paint gives many people headaches – paints, varnishes, and the various solvents we use to mix them and to clean up afterwards can be dangerous, and also present disposal problems. Oil-based paints in particular contain many hazardous chemicals, including heavy metals.

While all-natural paints are, at present, much more expensive than ordinary commercial brands, they should definitely be used in infants' and children's rooms. You'll be pleased by their light, slightly aromatic scent. As an intermediate step, choose water-based products and improve ventilation. Fresh air is more effective than heat in drying paint. If possible, allow a room to dry for several days before you move into it; paint baby's room well in advance of the birth.

Another option is to make your own paints. These include traditional water-based distemper and milk paint. Ingredients include sizing, whiting and artists' pigments. Some people love these because they give more interesting finishes and subtler colours than commercial paints. The most natural furniture finish is simple oil or wax, and traditional shellac is made from natural materials, not petrochemical products.

■Clean Up And Disposal

White spirits and other paint cleaners are hazardous and should be used with care. First, don't buy more than you need – if you use water-based latex paints you do not need white spirits as brushes can be cleaned with plain water. Second, after you've used an oil-based paint and cleaned your brushes in a jar of white spirits (don't leave them to soak), put the covered jar aside for several days. After the solids settle, pour the clear liquid into a new jar and save for the next project (if you're going to be using it as a paint thinner rather than as a brush cleaner, you may want to use an old coffee filter to remove any impurities remaining). The paint sludge in the bottom of the first jar can be disposed of (save it for hazardous waste collection, should your local authority run such a programme, or scrape it into the ordinary rubbish).

Experts believe that oil-based paints should be treated as hazardous waste and disposed of in separate sites, not be landfilled with ordinary domestic waste. The best solution is to use them up: buy what you need, and give any extras to a neighbour or charity, or help set up a paint exchange in your community. One US company is now processing and marketing recycled latex paint, in muted neutral colours at a modest price.

■Ecological Renovation

Anthropologist Paul Oliver estimates that over 95 per cent of the world's dwellings are self- or community-built, not designed by an architect and put up by a developer. This tradition died out long ago in most of Europe but an increasing number of people are now reviving some old homebuilding skills as they restore, renovate and extend their house. All houses need regular maintenance and as old buildings are turned to new uses renovation is increasingly common.

Improvements can make our homes more energy-efficient. Renovating an existing building is less damaging to the environment than building a new one, and there are many ways to reduce the impact of renovation while creating a healthier and more beautiful home.

RENOVATION IN A NUTSHELL

- Salvage as much as possible for reuse.
- Beware of toxic materials in what you remove.
- Use least toxic methods.
- Replace inefficient older windows.
- Fit insulation while you have the opportunity.
- Set up separate bins for recyclable materials.
- Choose new items made from recycled materials.

Salvage as much as possible for reuse. Window trim wood panelling, doors, floorboards, tiles and bricks, and framing timber can be removed carefully and set aside for reuse by you or someone else. Contractors don't like to do this because careful demolition takes longer, but you can certainly salvage materials when doing it yourself or you can handle certain stages of the demolition. Clean and store salvaged material – you might even be able to sell things you don't need yourself.

Beware of hazards in the materials you remove. Anything painted with lead paint should be disposed of rather than burned, and if you are stripping lead paint you should wear a respirator or high-quality dust mask. Other possible hazards include lead solder, asbestos (found in some floor and ceiling tiles), and wood treated with long-lasting pesticides.

Use least toxic methods as you work, choosing hand tools when you can and scraping surfaces by hand rather than using chemicals if possible. Wallpaper can often be removed with plain hot water.

Replace inefficient older windows, if your budget allows, with new high-performance thermally efficient windows. Most of these work through a combination of double or triple paned glass and tight sealing. This is a long-term energy saving investment, considerably less expensive and more attractive than double glazing. This is also a good time to improve wall and loft insulation.

Before you start a major renovation project, contact your local council, or Friends of the Earth, to find out what materials can be recycled in your area. They may be able to refer you to a charity that will welcome some of your discards. As you work, have separate bins or boxes to sort material for recycling or reuse: steel, aluminium, wood scraps, corrugated cardboard, insulation and wire.

Finally, complete the cycle by choosing new building products made from recycled materials. These include certain insulation materials, recycled plastic 'lumber,' various composites used for worktops and even recycled paint. These products are gradually coming on to the market – look for them and use them whenever you can.

7

ENERGY CHOICES

Our energy habits are wasteful and destructive, and they threaten many things we hold dear, but with the continually rising price of electricity and gas, as well as petrol, and tax changes and privatization, your main concern about energy may be whether you'll be able to afford as much as you need to maintain your standard of living.

The EU has, as part of an international effort to reduce carbon dioxide emissions and stabilize global warming, plans to devise a system of energy taxes, something the Worldwatch Institute in Washington DC has advocated for some years. This strategy would be to allow markets to operate unimpaired by quotas while encouraging investment in energy efficiency and renewable supplies, with a direct impact on carbon dioxide levels.

Before looking at the practicalities of home conservation, insulation and even simple solar energy, however, we need to consider the basic problems of energy use.

CLIMATE CHANGE

Fossil fuels – coal, oil and natural gas – provide most of the world's commercial energy. Supplies of these are limited (estimates range from 20 to 300 years for different fuels). When they are burned carbon dioxide (CO_2) is released – and this CO_2 is the primary cause of the 'greenhouse effect'. The amount of CO_2 in the atmosphere is now more than 15 per cent higher than in pre-industrial times and could easily double within the next 50–100 years. The Meteorological Office predicts a 5.2°C rise in global temperatures, which will lead to extensive flooding around the world.

CO_2 is transparent to incoming radiation but impedes the escape of heat (infra red radiation) from the earth. This heating effect is amplified by a roughly comparable amount of heating owing to a build-up of other trace gases (methane, CFCs and nitrous oxide). The precise effects of the expected rise in temperature are uncertain, but according to the Washington DC Worldwatch Institute, 'Climate change looms as the ultimate environmental threat. Its impact would be global and, for all practical purposes, irreversible.' The main impacts will be on weather, agriculture and global water levels.

No technical solution to this problem is known except reduced combustion of fossil fuels, which account for four-fifths of global energy use. Worldwide energy efficiency is the main way to limit the temperature rise to no more than 1°C, which would still mean serious consequences around the globe but would probably enable us to avoid the worst climatic effects.

The cutting down of tropical rainforests is also making a substantial contribution to the greenhouse effect, both because there are fewer trees to use available carbon dioxide and because unused plant material burned or left to decay when forests are cleared releases CO_2. Another suspected factor is a reduction in the oceans' phytoplankton caused by marine pollution.

ACID RAIN

We've all heard about acid rain. What is it? When fossil fuels are burned – to generate electricity, power our car engines or run the factories which produce steel – a number of chemicals are released, in addition to the carbon dioxide which is causing the greenhouse effect, and these cause acid rain.

Approximately 100 million tons of sulphur dioxide are released into the atmosphere each year. This sulphur forms a dilute sulphuric acid solution in rain water, and the resultant acid rain is killing plant and animal life in lakes across Europe and North America, has already damaged or destroyed more than one-fifth of Europe's forests, and the surfaces of buildings and historic monuments dissolve. Many lakes in Scandinavia and in the US are dead, completely empty of any aquatic life.

It is possible to filter the sulphur in a properly designed power station, but the current British government's policy has been to resist these changes – an attitude not appreciated by Norwegians, whose forests are being killed by the sulphur emissions from UK power stations.

NUCLEAR POWER

The nuclear industry continues to portray itself in a extensive advertising campaign as green, clean energy for the twenty-first century. The business community disagrees. The Confederation of British Industry (CBI) continues to be opposed to any new programme to build more nuclear power stations and has called for an end to government subsidies. It only reluctantly agreed to support a sell-off of the industry, expressing grave doubts about the economic viability of privatization.

The day-to-day health threat from nuclear power stations is discussed in Chapter 11, but it is interesting to note that even the Nuclear Installations Inspectorate is not happy with safety standards at a number of power stations. These problems are forcing the early closure of some stations, the cost of decommissioning is uncertain and there is still no solution to the problem of radioactive waste.

The disposal versus storage debate is a misnomer, as this waste (in Britain, an estimated 2 million m^3 by 2030) is not 'disposable'. The question is simply one of where it is to be stored, whether at processing stations, buried in land or in deep sea storage.

The government supported the nuclear power industry to the tune of some £220 million for 1993–4 (Department of Trade and Industry), while government research spending on renewable energy was only £25 million. These figures are better than those of a few years previously but the discrepancy remains enormous. Imagine if the 10 per cent surcharge on electricity bills in England and Wales which subsidizes Nuclear Electric, the so-called nuclear levy, was instead spent developing safe and sustainable sources of power, and investing in energy efficiency.

Nuclear power is being phased out in some countries and is at a standstill in the US, where no nuclear power stations have been ordered within the past decade and all orders since 1974 have been cancelled. Its 'technical, economic, and political problems now appear severe enough to rule out substantial expansion', according to the Worldwatch Institute.

THE OTHER ENERGY CRISIS

In the third world, the most serious energy crisis is the shortage of firewood. This has led to overcutting and deforestation, and causes soil erosion, flooding and food shortages. People in need of fuel burn animal dung and agricultural waste which could otherwise be used to enrich the soil.

Effective aid must take this into account. If you are wondering about where to give money to help with a current disaster in the third world, consider sending something to an organization like Intermediate Technology which is helping to develop things like efficient cooking stoves that can be made by the people who will use them from locally available materials.

HUMAN HEALTH

No one who lives or travels near busy roads can be unaware of the air pollution caused by our vehicles, and the problem is compounded by emissions from power stations and industry. There are short-term effects on human health like emphysema, bronchitis, asthma (which now affects one in seven children) and upper respiratory disease. Deaths from these causes have been reduced considerably over the past 20 years, but there remains a second major health concern, human cancers caused by air pollutants.

Another useful point to consider is that 'Energy conservation could lead to more exercise, better diets, less pollution, and other indirect benefits to human health' (Worldwatch Paper 4, *Energy: the Case for Conservation*, 1976).

THE ENERGY-EFFICIENT HOME

Independent energy experts know that by making full use of presently available energy-saving technologies, global energy use could be stabilized immediately, allowing us time to switch to alternative fuel sources and enabling us substantially to avert the crises which threaten us. In fact they say it would be possible over time to provide sufficient energy for everyone throughout the world to enjoy the sort of standard of living we now have in Western Europe.

Super-efficient fridges, long-life lightbulbs and cars which can run at nearly 100 m.p.g. are some of the technologies they have in mind. Over the past two decades, appliance efficiency standards have been developing in the US, and by the year 2000 these are likely to have saved $28 billion worth of electricity and gas, and kept 342 million tons of carbon out of the atmosphere.

Our buildings are the most wasteful energy users in industrial countries. Changing our use of energy is one of the highest environmental priorities. Turning down the heat and insulating the attic may seem mundane, but these steps are important and architects are increasingly conscious of energy-efficient design. There are a number of model building projects around the country where energy use is as little as one-quarter of that in similar but conventionally built houses.

With good insulation, the right materials and careful orientation, remarkable savings are possible. Imagine cutting your fuel bill from £60 per quarter to £15, and cutting down on your contribution to carbon and sulphur in the atmosphere at the same time! Our extremely inefficient use of fossil fuels not only pollutes our air, but acidifies our lakes, toxifies our soil and makes us sick, and while cutting energy use is never going to be glamorous it directly benefits us and the world we live in. Individually, we can choose energy-efficient appliances and products. We can also start to adopt, in practice, the idea that ways of saving energy – 'negawatts' – are a better buy than energy generation.

CHOOSING YOUR FUELS

Using electricity for 'low-grade' energy such as domestic heating and hot water is exceedingly wasteful because it is produced in power stations which burn large quantities of coal or oil and are, at best, only 35 per cent efficient. An open coal fire, by contrast, is 20 per cent efficient (i.e. 80 per cent of the heat goes up the chimney) and a gas furnace is about 70 per cent efficient. When we heat by electricity we lose over 90 per cent of the fuel's primary energy because of the inefficiency of the transmission systems and electrical appliances – based on these figures, electricity is even less efficient than an open fire.

Electricity is suitable only for 'high-grade' energy needs: lights, powering electronic equipment and motorized appliances. Gas and coal, however, are the best fuels for space heating and hot water, which make up 80 per cent of home energy use. A well-designed, energy-efficient wood or coal-fired stove may be your best space heating option and they can certainly be pleasant to live with. A better source of energy for space heating is the sun, a renewable 'fuel'.

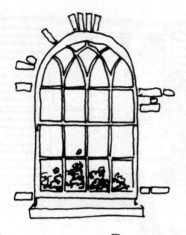

RENEWABLE SOURCES

The coal and oil supplies we are so rapidly using up were laid down millions of years ago, and once they are gone there won't be any more. Renewable energy sources, on the other hand, can be indefinitely sustained. There are a wide variety of potential energy sources: sunlight, wind, flowing water, wood and plants. These, too, have to be managed with care so as not to be used up more quickly than they replace themselves (that is, one would use only as much wood from a tree as grows each year).

The tapping of renewable sources of energy has made remarkable strides over the past decade, even without anything like the measure of support enjoyed by conventional and nuclear power supplies. They are particularly suitable for the small-scale, local projects recommended by many energy researchers. Small does not mean inefficient. In fact, huge electricity generating plants have turned out to be far less efficient than their creators envisaged back in the 1940s and 1950s. In the US small renewable energy projects are now able to sell power to the public utility companies.

Even urban homes can take advantage of the energy of the sun for heating (see 'Simple Solar Energy', below, p. 122) and very simple systems are available which will provide hot tap water throughout much of the year. Check with the Centre for Alternative Technology for details (see Sources).

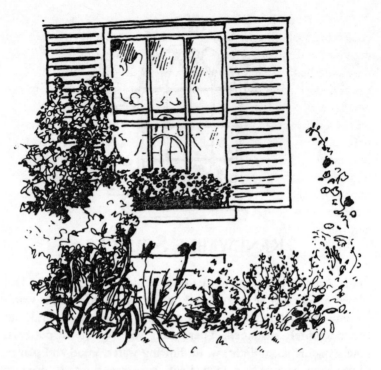

PRACTICAL STEPS YOU CAN TAKE

In the US, energy companies are responsible for increasing public awareness of the need for energy conservation, and they
provide free energy audits (or analyses) to customers. The financial incentive for the companies is the fact that conservation is
cheaper than building new power stations: companies invest in
'negawatts'.

But without professional guidance, you can still get an idea of
areas for improvement in your home. Analyse your electricity
and gas bills, look for opportunities to insulate and draughtproof.
The rest of this chapter consists of energy-saving ideas and techniques. You can take more specific action to help solve the
environmental problems caused by wasteful energy use than for
any other single problem discussed in this book. Many of the
actions are extremely easy and all of them will save you money.

As you read, note the ones you want to try. There are many books and publications available which give detailed advice on materials and methods. Your local library will have some, *Which?* magazine has frequent articles about cutting fuel bills, and the gas and electricity boards can offer advice. These suggestions do not depend on a switch to renewable energy sources or to new technologies; there are ways of making the best of whatever system you have now. (If you are planning to renovate or to build a new home, however, do some research into design and new systems that could save you even more money.) Energy conservation may be the easiest step to take in creating a green home – because you can judge your success so directly. The lower your fuel bills get, the better you're doing.

DRAUGHTPROOFING

1. Stuffed draught-excluders – those snake-shaped bolsters – are an easy and cheap way to prevent draughts under doors.
2. Fold newspaper into long, thick strips and use them to fill gaps between sash windows and frames (windows which you don't plan to open through the winter). Hold the strips in place while you shut the window.
3. Commercial draught strips are useful, but choose the more expensive, durable kind instead of adhesive foam, which disintegrates after a year or two and is hard to remove. Brass 'atomic strip', if you can find it, is durable and quite attractive.
4. Curtains can be nearly as effective as double-glazing at cutting draughts. The longer they are, the better (floor-to-ceiling are particularly good for draughtproofing).
5. Open doors as infrequently as possible in cold weather (put out the milk bottles when you let the cat in, for instance).

6. On doors that are used a lot, try to arrange some sort of airlock. The idea is to prevent gusts of wind blowing straight through the house when the door is opened. You do this by having two doors; the outside one is closed before the inside one is opened (or vice versa). This can be done fairly easily in a house or flat with a narrow front hall, by putting in an interior door (solid or glazed). A porch or small conservatory will serve the same function. (If your front door opens into a living room, you can at least increase comfort, although probably not save a great deal of heat, by creating an entry area with a large screen or room divider arranged to prevent direct draughts on people sitting in the room.)

7. Spring hinges ensure that frequently used doors stay closed.

8. Chimneys have to be well ventilated in order to draw properly (you can tell that you've over-insulated if your chimney stops drawing – you'll get a house full of smoke). But an unused fireplace can be very draughty. Either (a) install an efficient stove; (b) brick it up – incorporating air bricks as required; or (c) block it up with a fitted frame covered with board, with holes to allow some air through. Then you'll need half a dozen potted plants or a large vase of dried flowers on the hearth.

■Insulation

1. Fitted double-glazing is expensive, inflexible and resource intensive. *Which?* magazine says 'double-glazing does not save enough to be worth installing on cost criteria alone (thick curtains and insulating blinds are almost as effective)'. Secondary double-glazing (detachable in case of fire), however, can be installed fairly cheaply and even cheaper is plastic film fitted with a hairdryer. A more attractive and per-

manent solution is to use double-pane glass in existing window frames.

2. Heavy curtains are cheaper than double-glazing, easier to manoeuvre and look elegant. Look in auctions or you can make them yourself – the bigger and thicker, the better. Quilted curtains are also very warm. Curtains can also be used over doors and at the top of draughty stairs. You can buy special lining fabric, aluminium or plastic-coated, for extra insulation. Curtains should be shut as soon as it gets dark outside for maximum heat retention.

3. Shutters are even more effective than curtains and provide a good measure of security too. You can find appropriate ones from a salvage firm or get new ones made up by a joiner. There's no reason why you can't add shutters to modern windows.

4. Loft insulation has been well publicized as a means of cutting fuel bills and for some years there were grants available for this (they are now limited to people on low incomes). Use mineral fibre, vermiculite chips or cellulose fibre (made from recycled newsprint) rather than synthetic materials, and make sure that insulation goes over your cold water tank, to prevent it freezing.

5. Cavity wall insulation is suitable for some homes. Do not use urea-formaldehyde foam, which has been banned in the US because of its danger to health (more about formaldehyde on pages 94–95). Mineral fibre is a better ecological choice than polystyrene beads.

6. Hot water tanks need a warm jacket (like loft insulation, the pay-back period on this is only a couple of months). Get a large size and fit it over the old, thin one. You can also pad it with the same mineral fibre used in the loft, before putting the jacket on, and a layer of old blankets or clothes salvaged from the jumble sale bag make a cheap, additional layer of

insulation. Water pipes should be wrapped too.

7. Floors are insulated by carpeting and sheet flooring, but you
    can improve on this with thick fibre underlay, a layer of
    newspapers under the underlay or directly under linoleum
    (choose old-fashioned natural resin linoleum). Exposed sus-
    pended timber floors are best insulated with an under-floor
    layer, but this is a big job to tackle. Eliminate draughts by fill-
    ing cracks with an appropriate tinted filter (papier mâché
    works well).

8. Reflect heat with aluminium foil under non-vinyl wallpaper,
    and behind radiators and appliances, shiny side facing you
    (use a heavy duty wallpaper paste).

■Heating And Hot Water

1. Use a timer. Electronic programmers allow you different set-
    tings for different days, and to time heating and water
    separately.

2. Heat only the rooms you use, when you use them. This is
    standard advice, but in fact you may be better off with a dif-
    ferent approach – see below.

3. Fit thermostatic valves to radiators and use room ther-
    mostats. The hot water cylinder needs a thermostat too. Get
    family agreement as to acceptable temperatures!

4. Look for systems with spark ignition rather than a pilot light.
    These are safer (because the flame cannot blow out) and do
    not burn gas 24 hours a day.

5. Radiators should be placed on interior walls, contrary to the
    usual pattern – which is intended to warm draughts before
    they enter the room. Draughtproof your windows and this
    becomes unnecessary. If you have radiators on external walls,

at least paste sheets of aluminium foil (shiny side facing you) on to the wall behind them.

6. Shelves that are situated above radiators direct warm air into the room rather than allowing it to rise to the ceiling: a layer of aluminium foil on the underside of the shelf makes this more efficient (you can purchase ready-made deflective shelves).

7. If your ceilings are very high, consider building a platform area to take advantage of the warm air near the ceiling, and increase your living space at the same time. A ceiling fan or heat recycling pump will circulate the warm air.

8. Move your living room upstairs, at least in winter, to take advantage of rising heat. When installing a new central heating and hot water system, look at versions which run directly off the mains. They can be cheaper to run, give better water pressure (good in a flat if you want a shower) and mean that you do not need water tanks (thus gaining storage space).

9. If you have a hot water tank, lag it properly, and use the heat it still gives off for an airing cupboard.

10. Lower the temperature of your hot water until you can use it for a shower or bath without adding cold water. Many heaters are set to 140 but 120 is enough for most households.

11. Avoid letting hot water go down the drain, when possible. Allow bath and washing-up water to get cold before pulling out the plug – its heat is given off into the room.

■ Comfort Zones

More and more homes in the UK have central heating, but before you put in a centralized system you may want to consider the following points. What we really want is not a particular heating system, but a comfortable place to live and central heating has a number of disadvantages.

Many people complain of the stuffy, dry atmosphere in centrally heated rooms and compensate for this stuffiness with humidifiers (or wet towels hung over the radiators!). Winter colds and flu seem to increase when central heating is on because the dry air affects the protective membranes of the respiratory system.

According to the *National Trust Manual of Housekeeping*, 'In this country central heating has become perhaps the largest single factor in causing damage to the contents and even the structure of our houses.' A relative humidity (RH) of 50–60 per cent is ideal – for people as well as bookcases – but it sometimes drops as low as 20 per cent in centrally heated houses. The ideal situation is an even low temperature of not more than 60°F/15°C. The *Manual* also mentions that we should avoid Calor gas and paraffin heaters because they produce minute quantities of sulphur dioxide, forming an acid vapour which will harm furniture: indoor acid rain.

In her book *Healing Environments*, architect Carol Venolia discusses the way we have become engrossed in creating 'thermally stress-free environments' – central heating in winter and air-conditioning in summer – assuming that constant temperature is desirable, whereas this lessens sensory input and is actually bad for us, mentally and physically.

Everyone has a different comfort zone, depending on time of day, season and state of health, but in general the most comfortable heating for human beings is a combination of convected and radiant heat. Christopher Alexander suggests that this is biologically built into us by our evolution in the open air, with plenty of sunlight. Examples of this combination are sitting in warm sunshine on a mild spring day or in front of a glowing fire in a fairly cool room. Think of your own experiences and try to produce an environment that is as consistently satisfying as possible, without excessive dependence on central heating.

Your personal comfort depends on the rate at which your body loses heat to the air and this depends largely on the surface temperature of the objects around you. Although your body conducts some heat to the air around you, most of its heat is lost through radiation – just like a radiator. Radiation takes place through space, from one solid object to another, so the rate of radiation has to do mainly with the temperature of walls, floors and furniture, not the temperature of the air itself (which is what thermostats measure). Using plenty of natural, thermally neutral materials such as wood, cork and fabric – rather than brick and tile, enamelled steel and glass which heat and cool readily – will enable you to maintain a more even, comfortable environment.

The proper balance is a radiant temperature about 2° higher than the air temperature. This simply means keeping room temperature quite low (as the National Trust suggests), but having a heat source like a stove or an open fire, especially in rooms where people gather in cold weather. A fire provides a delightful focus to a room.

■ Staying Warm

1. How warm you feel depends on your metabolism, your body fat, your biological rhythms and on how much exercise you get. Do a little running on the spot to warm yourself up on cold mornings.

2. Hot food and drinks are a great help. And you can use a mugful of coffee or vegetable broth to warm your hands.

3. Dress with lots of layers. Tights or long underwear are good under trousers. Wool and cotton are warmer than synthetics, but it can be useful to wear a thin synthetic layer next to your skin when it's very cold, with a cotton shirt outside (and whatever collection of jumpers seems necessary). Any sweat 'wicks' through the synthetic fabric and into the natural material, where it slowly evaporates while the layer next to your skin stays dry. And remember to keep your feet warm.

4. Use good, old-fashioned warming methods like soft rugs to wrap up in when you are sitting at home in the evening.

5. In bed, a hot water bottle is very comforting. Recent studies on electric underblankets express concern about the effects of electromagnetic radiation (one newspaper report was titled 'Electric blankets in cancer enquiry'). Miscarriages are more common in couples who usually sleep with electric blankets.

6. Thick cotton flannel sheets make the bed feel warmer. A flannel duvet cover can be made from a pair of sheets. Flannel – or 100 per cent cotton – is soft and pleasantly absorbent in hot weather too. A wool blanket under the sheet seems to help the bed warm up.

7. Warm clothing at night certainly helps – socks, a sweater over your pyjamas, even a nightcap (most heat loss is from your head).

■Keeping Cool

As modern buildings do not have the more than adequate ventilation of traditional British homes, air-conditioning is on the increase in the UK, even though it cuts us off from natural light and air, and does not allow or encourage our bodies to adapt to heat. Changes in temperature are a form of natural stimuli which we need to stay tuned to the environment around us – to stay healthy, in fact. The need for it can be obviated by a number of simple architectural devices that are part of green home planning.

1. Dress for the heat in loose, light clothing. A sheer dress is more comfortable than tight shorts – think of a sari. Avoid synthetic fabrics. Cotton and linen may wrinkle, but you will be infinitely more comfortable.

2. Spray yourself with spring water, sprinkle water on your head, wet your clothes or go swimming.

3. Drink cool drinks. (Or hot ones, if you are one of those who believe that a cup of tea is cooling.)

4. Open windows at night and close them during the day. Keep the curtains closed too while sun is shining directly on the windows. Outdoor planting can provide welcome shade during warm summer months.

5. Ensure that there is plenty of air movement, either by cross-ventilation or an electric fan. A dampened curtain or sheet hung near a breezy window or in front of an electric fan will cool the air.

6. Use a hand fan – a collection of exotic fans is beautiful arranged on a wall, and you can offer them round to guests at a party.

■Appliances

Suggesting that we should be conscious of the energy we use doesn't mean giving up all our mod cons, but do think about just what you need to be able to live without too much hardship before you acquire more.

A dishwasher probably saves time for a large family that does a lot of entertaining and certainly keeps the kitchen a lot tidier, but there are sound arguments against having one. You need more crockery and miss out on companionable chats over the washing-up. Dishwashers require strong detergents (read the warning label) and use large amounts of hot water as well as considerable amounts of energy for drying. On the other hand, run on an economy cycle with full loads, a dishwasher can use less water than handwashing. If you use a dishwasher, look out for a phosphate- and chlorine-free washing powder, and cut the amount you use it to a minimum. Choose the economy setting and turn the machine off when it gets to the dry cycle – open the door and pull the racks out to air dry. The dishes are already hot so this takes very little time.

Christina Hardyment, author of *From Mangle to Microwave*, argues that supposedly time-saving appliances, and their manufacturers' substantial advertising budgets, have created impossibly high housekeeping standards – that they have, in fact, made women's lot harder, not easier (the same might be said of modern miracle cleaning products).

1. Think of any appliance as a long-term investment. Buy good quality models (check *Which?*), and keep them in working order by following manufacturers' instructions (except that you can halve the suggested amount of washing powder) and having them serviced regularly.

2. Do you really need a dishwasher/video machine/second television (or even first television)? If possible, borrow or hire one for a month or so, to see if you really make use of it.

3. If you can afford a new cooker with a self-cleaning oven, think about using the money to pay for some help instead.

4. Doing without a TV can free a surprising amount of time and maybe your mind too. Watch important programmes at a friend's house.

5. Look for equipment made of metal rather than plastic, which can release fumes, especially when heated, and tends to break. Try buying second-hand, through the adverts in the local paper or newsagents' window, or reconditioned models. Older models are often more solidly made, and as well as saving money you'll be keeping useful equipment in circulation, instead of on the scrap-heap. (Keep in mind that a high-quality new appliance with energy-saving features may be a better buy.)

6. While you want to make good use of your appliances, don't let having a food processor tempt you into blending/processing everything. Some chefs complain that food processors spoil the texture of food.

7. Look for hand-operated models. Carpet sweepers are great, especially if you like to give the main areas of wear a quick

going-over every day (carpets last longer if they are swept or vacuumed frequently).

8. A larder can expand your cold storage considerably (unrefined oils, wholegrain flours, seeds and nuts should be kept cool), so you may need only a small fridge.

■Fuel Combustion By-Products

It was better home insulation which led to awareness of the dangers of combustion by-products, which include formaldehyde, nitrogen dioxide, sulphur dioxide, and a host of other vapours and gases, because in a well-insulated house they build up more than in a traditional draughty British home. For people sensitive to petrochemicals and those with health problems (including emphysema, asthma and angina), this can be a matter for concern.

Be especially careful to ensure that gas appliances have plenty of ventilation while in operation. They must be correctly adjusted in order to burn efficiently; if they burn inefficiently there will be unnecessary fumes given off. Your gas company can provide advice and service – send for the leaflet listed in Sources.

■Ventilation

It's no good insulating so well that bad smells, solvent fumes and moisture in the air have nowhere to go. A high tech, super-insulated building will need mechanical ventilation and indoor air pollution control will be essential. Avoiding toxic chemical products is going to be all the more important as we continue to improve building standards.

Extractor fans in the bathroom and kitchen can be automatically controlled by a 'dew stat' (bathroom fans generally have a timer). Opening a window a little bit is an alternative, as long as you remember to close it as soon as the moisture or smell you want to get rid of has cleared.

In the summer a small ceiling fan helps to keep the place cool, and in winter it circulates the warm air which would otherwise rise to the top of the room and stay there. More elaborate devices for circulating warmed air around the house are available too, such as David Stephens' (Practical Alternatives) VertiVent (see Sources).

■ Condensation

Internal damp is usually combated by turning up the heat, or by opening a door or window, both wasteful solutions! In centrally heated homes the air is often too dry, but some people fight a continual battle with damp. Condensation occurs when warm, moist air comes into contact with cold surfaces – when you turn the heating on in a cold house, for example. To avoid this:

1. use natural materials and fabrics (they absorb moisture and slowly release it back into the air);

2. cut the amount of water which gets into the air – cover cooking pots and don't dry clothes inside;

3. constant low heating can cost no more than occasional (morning and evening) heating and has the advantage of eliminating the main cause of condensation, by keeping surfaces and air at a fairly constant temperature.

■ Kitchen

1. Use an automatic switch-off electric kettle and heat only as much water as you need. Upright kettles make it possible to boil a single cup of water, but there is some concern over the fact that they are made of plastic, minute traces of which will inevitably dissolve into the water. Scale deposits will make your kettle less efficient, so clean with a strong vinegar solution from time to time. Filtering water – see Chapter 10, p. 166 – can remove the minerals which cause scale.

2. Put extra boiling water from the kettle into a thermos for later or use it to start soaking a pan of beans. This is a good budget move if you use filtered water for drinks and cooking.

An even easier way to keep a constant supply of hot water is to boil a full kettle and put a heavy towel over it after you have used what you need (same principle as a tea cosy).

3. Improve your health and save energy by eating more raw food, salads and fresh fruit.

4. Cover cooking pots to cut cooking time and save energy (you know, a watched pot never boils – put the lid on).

5. Let the fire fit the pan: flame licking up the side of a small saucepan is wasted. Try not to turn the grill on for a single piece of toast.

6. Use a pressure cooker (stainless steel rather than aluminium) to cut cooking time drastically. This is useful for beans you haven't remembered to soak.

7. Fill the oven. For example, bake a pan of apples on the lower shelf while a nutloaf – or joint of beef – is cooking, then put in a tray of meringues before turning the oven off and leave them overnight.

8. Cut vegetables, including potatoes, into small pieces: they cook much more quickly.

9. When preparing foods which take a long time, cook more than you need and save the rest for another meal. Cooked beans and grains keep for about a week in the fridge, and are excellent in salads.

10. A tiered steamer will do several vegetables at once, and you can use the bottom pan of a double boiler to simmer eggs or steam rice while you stir a curry sauce in the top.

11. For hot food, there's the option of slow cooking with a hay-box; a pot of stew or soup, or even porridge, is put into a box packed with hay which works like a vacuum flask to maintain

the heat. You can build an urban version with some leftover polystyrene packing, as long as you ensure that there is a good layer of newspaper or towelling between it and the hot pan.

12. Chest freezers are more efficient than upright models, though less convenient to use. If you have a freezer, defrost regularly and try to keep it full. Keeping it outside, in a garage or cellar, cuts energy costs, or you can put foil on the wall behind it to reflect waste heat into the room.

■Laundry

1. Wash full loads, and keep the cycles as short and cool as possible. Clothes can be rinsed in cold water, but a hot wash is probably preferable to using large amounts of detergent. If possible, let the machine fill with hot water heated by your gas system, rather than allowing it to heat electrically in the machine.

2. In dry weather, even in winter, hang clothes outside to dry (they'll smell wonderful) or on clothes drying racks indoors; if necessary finish in the airing cupboard or tumble dry for a few minutes.

3. According to *Which?*, a spin dryer can halve the time and energy needed to tumble dry a load of clothes, even after they have been spun in a washing machine. It makes drying clothes on racks much faster too.

4. It's all to the good if you can manage without your own washing machine at home. Communal laundry rooms are common in American apartment buildings.

5. Iron in bulk rather than one piece at a time for more efficient use of heat and of your time; use a heat reflective cover or cut a piece of aluminium foil to fit under your ironing board cloth cover.

6. Run automatic dryer loads back to back, while the dryer drum is hot.

■Lighting

One of the simplest steps in creating a green home is to install low-energy lightbulbs. They are initially expensive – you may want to replace ordinary lightbulbs gradually – but save a substantial amount of money in the long run. In addition, according to the Worldwatch Institute, every compact fluorescent bulb you use will save 180 kilograms of coal and keep 130 kilograms of carbon out of the atmosphere.

Switch to low-wattage bulbs where only a small amount of light is needed, in hallways, for example. Friends of mine with a new baby switched to 25 and 40-watt bulbs upstairs because it was pleasanter for night feedings, and found that the soft lighting also made getting up in the morning less of a shock to the system, though they did occasionally find themselves at the tube station in one brown and one navy sock. Always make sure you have enough light for safety and to avoid eye strain.

Light provides a certain measure of security, both on the street and at home. Use sufficient lighting to deter burglars, but put lights on a timer and use low-energy bulbs. Security lights which come on only if someone approaches the house no doubt save a little energy, too.

■Computers

Computers are becoming increasingly common at home, whether you have an office there or not, and while they are fairly small consumers of energy compared to heat-producing appliances, their ubiquitousness means reducing their energy use is important. Computer systems are thought to account for 5 per cent of total commercial energy use, but computers sit unused for long periods of time and many commercial systems are left to run 24 hours a day.

The major computer manufacturers are now producing PCs with a variety of energy-saving features. If you're buying a new machine, ask about green models. A few companies have begun making machines with recycled plastic components, reduced packaging, designed for easier recycling at the end of the machine's life, smaller components and monitors that meet demanding Swedish specifications for radiation (see Sources).

But you should not purchase a new PC simply to have a more energy-efficient model. Already, the information revolution is substantially increasing waste. The continual 'upgrading' of technology is expected to send 150 million PCs to landfill within the next five years. This waste is one of the unavoidable results of the pace of technological advance.

The computer industry has had a reputation for being clean because its plants are set in pristine parklike plazas, with no smoke stacks or noisy production lines. But the Silicon (Santa Clara) Valley in California has the highest concentration of Superfund sites in the US. The Superfund is a national toxic site clean-up programme monitored by the government and, apart from military bases, high technology manufacturing sites are its major focus.

Combination hardware and software devices are being developed to automatically 'power down' your computer when not in use. A conventional screen saver programme is intended to save wear on the screen, but the monitor still produces radiation and wastes electricity. It is possible to fit an inexpensive unit that will switch the screen itself off (see Sources for listings).

A few computer companies, under pressure from governments in the US and Japan, accept old computers for recycling parts and material, while non-profit groups and schools are often delighted to accept older PCs as gifts.

While these suggestions apply to the home office and game computers, you can also suggest that your company applies them. A green computer policy will save money and create a good image for the company with customers and employees.

■ Simple Solar Energy

If you are itching for a new DIY project you could tackle something like solar panels or a wind generator, but the simplest, cheapest form of renewable energy available to all of us is 'passive' solar heating. This means making maximum use of the sunlight that falls on your home.

1. Orientation is the most important factor – see Chapter 12 for more on this.

2. Have large south-facing windows and smaller ones in north-facing rooms to avoid excessive heat loss there.

3. Leave curtains open throughout the daylight hours, but close them promptly when it gets dark.

4. Don't use net curtains, especially on south-facing windows.

5. Remember that dark colours absorb sunlight (and heat), while light colours reflect it.

6. Take advantage of the thermal inertia of building materials. A brick floor will absorb heat from the sun during the day and give it off through the evening, just as a brick garden wall is perfect for espaliered fruit trees because of the way it retains warmth.

7. Conservatories are an ideal source of passive solar heat, and can make a substantial contribution towards warming your home, as well as providing an extra room (estate agents also consider them one of the best ways to add value to your property). If you are a gardener, consider a conservatory as a greenhouse built against the house. Choose a south or west-facing site if possible, out of the wind (you can plant windbreak trees or shrubs). Double glass will help to eliminate any need for heating, and you'll need blinds and ventilation for hot weather.

David Stephens, long a proponent of alternative energy and conservation, is in the process of building a solar village in Wales. For referral to an architect able to guide you in more substantial renovation, contact the Ecological Design Association.

8

OUT AND ABOUT: HOW WE GET AROUND

The car dominates our way of life so profoundly that it is difficult to see clearly how it affects our lives, our health and the health of our society. Car ownership is one of the statistical measures of a society's affluence and increases in mobility are generally considered a desirable thing; mobility is equated with independence.

In 1994, over 1.5 million cars were registered for the first time. In spite of the fact that most people do not drive regularly, over 99 per cent of the national transport budget is devoted to the automobile. The automobile is having a calamitous effect on our environment but we seem to be turning more than ever towards car ownership. As a result, UK traffic is expected to increase by 20–40 per cent over the next decade – an appalling thought. Instead of clinging to the 'independence' cars give us, we should be thinking about these environmental and social issues in planning the transport of the future.

The result of our dependence on the automobile has been

aptly termed urban thrombosis ('vessel blockage'). This blockage is inevitable as long as driving is encouraged by the building of new roads, tax concessions to companies and the neglect of public transport as a matter of public policy. Individually, we need to rethink the way we use our cars, recognizing that over emphasis on this particular form of transport is lowering the quality of life for everyone. All of us suffer the effects of traffic to some extent, but it is often people who do not own cars who suffer most from heavy traffic and badly planned traffic schemes: children, elderly and disabled people, and mothers pushing prams.

Rather than plan for more cars, and design towns and shopping centres that force more and more people to have them, we should be planning towns that have healthy mixed transportation and areas that are not dependent on cars. Local shops, post offices, hospitals and schools increase a sense of community identity, lessen our need to travel long distances for basic facilities and make life easier for the many people who do not drive.

POLLUTION

As we saw in Chapter 7 the burning of fossil fuels, including petrol, has a range of serious environmental consequences – from acid rain to global climate change. Car engines, which account for about one-third of our annual fossil fuel consumption, also affect the air, through emissions of nitrogen oxide, carbon monoxide, hydrocarbons and sulphur dioxide as well as, even today, lead.

Most of us have felt the effects of these pollutants while waiting for a bus by a busy road or while stuck in a traffic jam. Headaches and smarting eyes and throat are common complaints, but long-term damage is far more serious, and ranges from respiratory problems like bronchitis and asthma to lung cancer. Research shows a much increased rate of leukaemia among people exposed to high levels of benzene, and Italy has proposed legislation to cut benzene levels in petrol. In the US, petrol stations have posted warnings about the hazards of petrol fumes and most petrol pumps have special caps to reduce evaporation.

ILL HEALTH AND STRESS

Cars are bad for us and not only because they cause air pollution. Equally important to our health is the fact that driving requires no physical effort. Our bodies are atrophying for lack of use. Some of us make up for this with regular exercise, but many people do not. Cutting down on car use – switching to cycles or foot for short journeys – could substantially improve human health.

Traffic congestion is a source of irritation and stress to drivers. In the US there have been a number of cases of angry motorists drawing guns on each other. Many people will go to almost any length to avoid traffic jams, even when this means using residential streets, threading through the back roads favoured by professional commuters.

Traffic noise is an insidious pollutant, perhaps most striking in its absence – when, for example, snow blocks the roads. The problem grows as traffic grows and influences even rural villages. Many people hesitate to open windows because of the roar of traffic outside their homes, while others have trouble getting to sleep at night because of cars and motorcycles zooming past. Goods lorries with diesel engines are largely responsible for unacceptable noise levels and emit eight times more smoke than the equivalent vehicle run on petrol.

SOCIAL REPERCUSSIONS

Cars are inherently dangerous: they are large, heavy objects which travel at high speeds in close proximity to pedestrians and cyclists. Only careful road and town planning, with restrictions on cars in residential and shopping areas, and an overall reduction in traffic volume, can alleviate this problem.

Cars, roads and car parks take up approximately one-third of all land in an average city. Congestion on the roads makes crossing more difficult for pedestrians and parked cars frequently block the pavement. Motorways cut swathes through large stretches of the country, obliterating everything in their path.

Many valuable and beautiful wildlife sites have been destroyed already, and more are on the chopping block at the Department of Transport.

In addition, local identity is seriously affected by heavy traffic. The more traffic there is in a particular area, the less likely are residents to know their neighbours and to think of it as home territory. Motor vehicles have taken over 'common land' – the space between houses and workplaces which used to act as a meeting ground. There is speculation that this may explain the rise of 'agoraphobia' (literally, fear of the 'agora', or market place), a psychological disorder in which sufferers are afraid to go outside for any reason at all; we no longer feel that we have a right to be in public places.

There are five principles to keep in mind if you are trying to improve the traffic situation in your area.

1. Improve public transportation and increase public awareness of the benefits of using it. Schools could get involved in a campaign.

2. Reduce the amount of traffic on residential streets: make them unattractive to rat-running motorists by adjusting traffic priorities at junctions, and installing road closures and chicanes. These schemes help to limit traffic to local residents, and careful planning to include plenty of trees and shrubs, which help muffle noise and improve the air, can make streets far more pleasant for residents.

3. Reduce vehicle speeds with traffic humps, width restrictions and street 'furniture' such as chicanes to slow cars down and make roads safer for everyone.

4. Install special cycling facilities: exempt cyclists from some one-way restrictions and road closures, as well as providing special cycle paths and turning lanes. This will encourage more people to cycle, as will increased safety from reduced and slower traffic.

5. Special pedestrian facilities: wider and higher pavements increase pedestrians' security, and a pavement extended straight across the road at a junction forms a clear pedestrian crossing and a traffic hump for motorists. Special footpaths and pedestrian shopping areas are other ways to improve towns for people on foot.

WOMEN AND TRANSPORT

Transportation is a particularly acute problem for women, who make shorter and more varied journeys than men, and generally have more to carry. Only one-third of British women drive, compared to two-thirds of British men, and far fewer have access to a car during the day.

Safety is a worry, particularly at night. Transport planning tends to ignore the special problems faced by women while staff cuts and poor design of public transport facilities – bad lighting and isolated staircases and subways – make women more vulnerable and therefore less likely to go out at all.

Cycle routes and special provisions for pedestrians are all the more important to women, particularly if they are escorting small children. Cycling is a lovely way to get around with a child (much faster than walking and ideal for local journeys), but unsafe road conditions deter most parents.

PUBLIC TRANSPORT

When one reads that a majority of people are travelling to work in cars – at a higher energy cost per mile than an aeroplane – it is all too easy to blame them for taking this route. There is, of course, individual choice involved (as well as social pressure), but it is not realistic to think that people are going to turn *en masse* to public transportation until governments put money into improving services. And there isn't a question of the money being there: millions are poured into the building of new roads. Government expenditure on public transport is called a 'subsidy', while money spent on more and bigger roads is not. The social and ecological costs of car travel are not yet being taken into account in traffic planning, the road lobby is powerful and better public transport is dismissed as uneconomic.

We need better bus and train services. By better I mean more reliable, faster, cleaner, safer and more comprehensive. Both city and country dwellers need a good public transport network. The closure of rural bus routes and train lines has left people in many villages and country areas isolated, or increasingly (and unnecessarily) dependent on cars.

We should support public transport, with our votes and by using it whenever we can. Join public pressure groups like Sustrans (Sustainable Transportation), Transport 2000 and Friends of the Earth, as well as any local association which campaigns on traffic issues. (An intriguing point for drivers to consider is that the best way to speed up car travel is to improve public transport.)

Using public transport requires somewhat different planning than travel by car, and the following ideas may make you more likely to choose to take the bus or train.

1. Set aside a shoebox for timetables and maps, and go out of your way to assemble a complete collection (these should be much more readily available). Libraries, town halls and police stations often have some, and bus garages and tube stations should be able to provide the full range. Put information numbers in a prominent place by the telephone and write them on the top of your shoebox. There may also be a number you can dial to get up-to-the-minute information on cancellations and delays.

2. Get whatever reduced price fares or cards you are entitled to. British Rail has a wide range of travelcards, and there are various concessionary tickets available for buses and the Underground. They are great incentives to use public transport, for weekend outings as well as shopping.

3. Get details of last buses, trains and night buses for your area.

The number of a reliable minicab service won't go amiss either.

4. Think about the personal benefits of not driving: time to read, doze or meditate, with no worries about parking or about having a drink.

5. Allow yourself enough time, so you can catch the right train without killing yourself with a last-minute dash to the station. This is a hard habit to get into if you are used to stepping out of the door into a car. A book is invaluable when waiting for a delayed train.

6. A shopping trolley or a rucksack and an easily collapsible pushchair will make all the difference if you have to manage large parcels or a small child.

7. Working on flexitime makes it possible to travel off-peak, avoiding packed buses and trains, and sometimes saving money too.

■ Tips For Rural Dwellers

1. Think about transport when you choose a new home.

2. Combine recreational walks with practical errands.

3. Patronise local shops to keep them going.

4. Form a car pool.

5. Use whatever public transport you have – write letters to your local paper and MP to emphasize its importance.

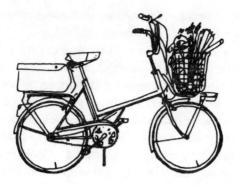

ON YOUR BIKE

Cycling is a convenient, efficient and enjoyable way to get around. It's much faster than walking and faster than driving in many cities, eminently suited to short journeys. But there's no doubt that a mass of metal threatens you every time you venture out. In a collision, the cyclist is always the one at risk. But a transport strategy giving high priority to bicycles would change everything. How wonderful it would be to have separate bicycle paths, plenty of marked bicycle routes and counter-flow lanes on one-way streets. In the long term, measures like these are essential to getting lots of people on to bicycles, which the Worldwatch Institute calls 'vehicles for a small planet'.

There are some places where people do function without cars. On Sark, in the Channel Islands, visitors are charmed to find that everyone gets around on foot or bicycle; in Denmark ten times as many journeys are made by bicycle than in Britain (20 per cent compared to our 2 per cent); in Amsterdam, where the climate is no better than ours, a third of journeys are made by bicycle.

Cyclists can be far more flexible than drivers and alternative routes, using quieter residential roads, make travelling less stressful, safer and faster. Friends of the Earth can put you in touch with a local cycling group, many of which produce maps to share advice on good routes. If you're commuting, you'll soon find out where the traffic bottlenecks are and learn to avoid roads strewn with broken bottles. Sometimes parks have marked cycle paths.

An undervalued benefit of travelling by bicycle is how easy it is to stop and start (unlike travel by car or bus).

Getting ready to cycle seems like preparing for a demolition derby or worse. Instead of being a carefree family activity, in urban areas it is an act of courage and defiance to face the roads each morning. Some drivers behave appalling badly to bike riders and the rest seem oblivious. The more people there are who cycle the safer cyclists will be. We need a higher profile – in the press and in drivers' eyes, so they get used to looking out for us.

Many people wonder whether the exercise and transport benefits of bicycling are not outweighed by the stress of travelling in traffic and the damage that exhaust fumes do to your lungs, not to mention your face, which gets rosy but filthy. Cyclists are especially vulnerable to smoke particulates because they are breathing deeply and some choose to wear masks. But the exercise makes you fit and therefore less likely to suffer from other health complaints.

■Children

Cycling is the ideal way for older children and teenagers to get around. Walking is slow and not an option for many people because of distances, public transport can be inconvenient for local journeys and driving children around takes up astonishing amounts of many parents' time. One study found that 24 per cent of the car journeys made by families with children under the age of 15, able-bodied 13 year olds as well as small children, were escort journeys, to and from school, sports activities, and music lessons or to friends' houses. It's no surprise that our children don't get enough exercise.

Safe bike routes are even more important for children than for adults. Campaign for bikes-only routes, support Sustrans' plan to develop a 5000-mile network of cycle paths in Britain, and sit down with your children to work out routes to frequent destinations. Ride them together once or twice to assess your youngster's skill and concentration.

If you use a bicycle for local shopping, get a childseat for small children (up to 40 lb). You can even buy a child-sized helmet.

Some parents use a tricycle or a trailer seat, which is very practical for shopping too.

■ Your Bicycle

If you're a new cyclist, buy a second-hand bike. You may want to move up to a fancier model when you get hooked and start planning trips through the Dales, but any bicycle in decent condition will manage journeys around town.

Find a shop for repairs and accessories. These places can be intimidating, full of athletic young staff wandering around in cycling sweatshirts and funny black shorts. Take a deep breath and explain that you intend to use your bicycle for commuting/shopping/touring or whatever, have so much to spend and need some specific help. You're looking for friendly, intelligent assistance. Make some notes and compare not only price but the quality of information you get. Do they talk about the cotterless cranks without explaining that this means the bits the pedals go on? What about guarantees, accessories and service policies?

An old-fashioned upright bike is practical around town and no one is likely to steal it. An alternative is the mountain bike. These sturdy conveyances are designed to cope with any terrain. City versions are slightly less rugged but their thick, heavy-tread tyres can handle roadways strewn with fragments of broken glass and death-dealing potholes better than a touring bike's narrow wheels. They are also good for going up and down kerbs.

A lightweight bike is easier to carry up and down stairs, but quality matters a lot more than lightness. At low speeds, up to about 14 m.p.h., weight matters more than air resistance, but the difference between a heavy and a light bike is only a small proportion of your combined weight. You're probably not worried about trimming ten seconds off your home-to-work speed.

Make sure the bike fits you and adjust the seat to the correct height. A rule of thumb is that with the saddle half extended on its pin, you should be able to touch the ground with both feet, without being on teetering tiptoe. This is important for back and knees, as well as for speed.

MAINTENANCE

- Get a repair kit and a spare inner tube. You may want to carry the kit and a small tyre pump with you.
- Good lights and reflective gear are essential if you will be riding in the dark. A helmet can save your life.
- Decide what you are going to do about rain, in advance. The right gear makes it easy to cope with light showers. Wear reflective clothing: really bad weather not only makes roads slippery but makes you far less visible to drivers.
- Fit a plastic flap at the bottom of your front mudguard to keep feet dry and clean.
- Good locks are essential – ask about the newest development at your bike shop.
- Find a secure place to lock your bike: parking meters and stout metal railings are ideal, and now and then you'll find a bicycle rack.
- Check tyre pressure weekly. Check tyres for fragments of glass, and tighten all nuts and bolts, too. Tune in to your bike so that when something isn't quite right, you hear it. A regular monthly tune-up – ten minutes on a Sunday afternoon – will make a big difference in reliability. (*Richard's New Bicycle Book* will take you through most maintenance procedures.)

■Cycling Gear

Cycling can be rough on shoes, even if you don't use toeclips, and office shoes may not give you sufficient grip on the pedals for safety or speed. Carry office shoes or stick them into a desk drawer at night.

Buy reflective bands or clips for your trouser legs, or make do with rubber bands. Tucking trouser legs into your socks doesn't look very elegant, but it does the trick. A bicycle chain can chew through expensive fabric in seconds so use a chain guard for commuting. Skirts are hard to manage on a bicycle and can be dangerous.

If you commute to work, perspiration is almost certain to be a problem during warm weather. Bicycling in town also gets clothes dirty. If you can change when you get to work, wear a riding ensemble (t-shirt, shorts and a pair of trainers) and carry your work clothes. Get into the office early to change – you'll look fresh and rosy when everyone else turns up.

If you can't change on arrival, wear as light a shirt as possible and open a few buttons while you are cycling. You may have to wipe down with damp paper towels in the WC. A fresh shirt, rolled or folded inside your saddlebag or left in a desk drawer, is good insurance.

A few lucky people work for companies like the Body Shop that provide changing and shower facilities.

WALKING

Most people in the world travel on foot because that is the only means of transport available to them, but many car owners never walk anywhere. Walking can be a great pleasure. You notice changes in the trees, watch the restoration being done on a dilapidated but beautiful old house, enjoy the tangy scent of newly turned earth or the luxurious smell of a bank of honeysuckle. The fresh air and light are good for your body, and walking gives you time to think, a precious commodity in our hectic lives.

Are we really so short of time that we cannot walk? Travelling by car frequently means fighting through heavy traffic, finding somewhere to park and walking to our actual destination. This is a matter of perspective: some people won't walk five minutes to buy a pint of milk but will spend ten minutes parking and walking from the car to the shop.

Country dwellers have the advantage here when it comes to pleasant places to walk, but even in urban and suburban areas it is possible to find interesting routes that keep you clear of the traffic and noise of the main roads, and offer a look at another

Britain. Wildlife groups have helped to turn abandoned railway lines into attractive pedestrian and cycle paths, as well as being preserves for many wild creatures, and in the 1990s Sustrans is working to build a national network of paths for cyclists and walkers. These include routes through the centres of major cities as well as routes in the countryside. Contact Sustrans for local information and to see what you can do to help promote sustainable transport where you live.

Brisk walking is nearly as good as jogging for your heart and for losing weight, so many people now walk for fitness. Not just a 5-minute stroll down to the sweet shop, but a vigorous 30 or 40 minutes – you might even be able to walk to work!

A small backpack is more practical than carrying a bag. And comfortable shoes are essential. Personal security is a thorny question and one which women face continually. If in doubt, do not walk (get a bus or minicab or ask a friend for a lift – and a few areas have special late-night women's lift services). For a day out, a compass is a good idea, in addition to maps, rain gear, proper boots, water and snacks.

Recreational walking ranges from an afternoon jaunt in the country (take a train to one station and travel home from another) to walking holidays. Britain has an incredible range of footpaths, though to find all of them you'll need to get good at navigating by Ordnance Survey maps. The Ramblers' Association is campaigning to preserve and protect the public's right of access to Britain's footpaths, because in some places it is being eroded by resistance and neglect on the part of property owners and local councils.

Even small children can cover a reasonable distance in a day, with plenty of pauses to examine beetles, and discuss the life and death of birds. For inspiration, read Dervla Murphy's *Where the Indus is Young* – the Irish travel writer took her five-year-old daughter walking in the Himalayas one winter. Babies and toddlers can travel in a sturdy back pack.

WHY DRIVE?

There are specific reasons people choose to drive. Infrequent or inconvenient public transport is one. Some people hate crowds. Others feel that riding on a bus is somehow demeaning. It may be raining, you may be late and you may not feel safe outside after dark.

But maintaining a car is time-consuming and expensive. If you don't have a car, is this a conscious choice or are you simply waiting until you pass a driving test or can afford the monthly payments? Taking taxis occasionally and hiring a car a couple of times a year works out considerably cheaper than keeping your own vehicle.

If you didn't have a car, how much extra time would you have to spend walking to the bus stop or the station? Perhaps 20 minutes a day, enough to keep you in reasonable shape. Another possibility is using a moped or motorbike, which use little fuel, do not add much to traffic congestion and are easy to park. (Motorcycles can also be noisy and dangerous, and leave you exposed to the elements just like a cyclist, but without the advantage of getting some exercise.)

■Driving As If People Mattered

If you have a car and never go anywhere without it, the first step towards increasing your awareness of pedestrian problems is to spend an hour or two walking around your own area. There are always a few places where it is virtually impossible for pedestrians to cross and other places where people hover in the middle of a busy road, waiting for a gap in the traffic. Apart from supporting local and national pressure groups to improve traffic conditions for everyone, there are a number of things drivers can do immediately to make the roads safer and pleasanter.

▶ Don't drive alone. Try car-pooling to work if you cannot use public transport, share driving the children to school and why not do your weekly shopping with a friend?

▶ Never drink and drive (what could be more obvious?) and be careful about drinking and cycling, too, especially if you have to cycle home through heavy traffic, where you need fast reflexes and all your faculties.

▶ Slow down. At 15 m.p.h. (25 km/hour), there is only 3 per cent chance of death for a pedestrian hit by a car, while at 40 m.p.h. (65 km/hour) the chance rises to 90 per cent. Men who get a buzz from driving fast should find another way of exhibiting their virility.

▶ Don't let common courtesies disappear when you get behind the wheel. Let people cross the street, slow down when there are children about and do not rev your engine to hurry pedestrians at a crossing. Stop when the lights turn yellow instead of streaking through, especially when there is someone waiting to cross. A calmer driving style will be good for your blood pressure – and bank balance!

▶ Learn to drive well. This means handling the vehicle, paying attention to what's going on and staying alert. Passing the driving test does not make you a good driver. (Friends of the Earth wants the driving test made more stringent and suggests regular testing of drivers rather than a lifetime licence.)

▶ Don't get angry at pedestrians or cyclists just for being there. Watch out when you open your car door, or reverse across the pavement, instead of assuming they will always look out for you.

▶ Don't be bullied by other drivers into driving too fast or dangerously.

▶ Slow down to 20 m.p.h. in residential districts (including your own). Even lower maximum speed limits are in force in some continental cities, and it is an easily adopted traffic calming measure.

▶ Get involved with your local residents' group and offer to work on traffic issues.

EMISSIONS

The EU has said that Britain must either develop a lean-burn engine, with low levels of emissions, or fit all new cars with catalytic converters. The UK decided on the new type of engine. Then the EU brought in legislation that says all cars produced after 1993 had to have a catalytic converter anyway.

The lean-burn engine may be a better option in Britain. Lean-burn engines are more efficient than engines with catalytic converters because the catalytic converter does not work well in a cool climate: a car has to do a considerable number of miles before the catalytic converter gets hot enough to work. They work fine in California, but not so well in the UK. Catalytic converters are expensive to fit to older cars and not all models can take them.

While lead-free petrol is now common, the problem of lead emissions has not been solved. Lead in petrol has two functions.

1. It allows the fuel to burn properly when the engine compresses it – raising the 'octane' – and thereby prevents 'knocking', which would damage the engine. When lead is removed, other octane improvers maintain this quality of petrol.

2. It forms a thin, tan-coloured coating on the valves which let the exhaust out of the engine. This stops them from getting worn – so-called 'valve seat recession'. If lead is reduced this protection becomes less effective in susceptible older engines. Most cars built since 1980 can run without lead since they have harder valve seats which wear less anyway (consult your manufacturer for specific details).

Older cars can be protected by using leaded petrol for one tank in three, as the lead remains on the valves for quite a time. The faster and hotter the engine runs, the more quickly the protective lead coating disappears, so drive sedately. Better yet, have your car converted to run on lead-free petrol. This involves replacing the valves and valve seats with the modern, hard variety, and is likely to cost about £200 for the average family saloon. Every manufacturer has an advisory service – ring your local dealer for more information.

WHEN YOU BUY A CAR

The lifespan of any car can be greatly extended by good maintenance and, most of all, by rust prevention. Some 1 million cars are junked every year. Since the manufacture of a car requires a large input of both energy and raw materials, keeping them alive is ecologically sound – buying a new one every time you have paid for the old one is not.

An important step in lengthening the life of your car is to spray on a thick coating of underseal (available from car accessory shops), after a thorough cleaning with a jet wash. This dries to form an impermeable layer and only needs to be touched up every three to four years. (New cars may come with this already done; check in your manual to see when a new coating will be needed.)

When you do buy, think about these points.

▶ Look at second-hand cars and get impartial advice if you feel you cannot judge yourself. Major problems with cars generally show themselves in the first 20,000 miles, so a second-hand car can be a better bet than a new one – and much cheaper.

▶ Get a car you like and will be happy to drive for many years. Buy the right size for your family and your frame. *Which?* gives useful advice.

▶ Look for low-pollution features. A car which gets good mileage means reduced running costs and fewer pollutants being pumped into the atmosphere.

▶ Do not choose a diesel engine – these are sometimes advertised as ecologically sound, but the fact is they produce far more particulant pollutant than standard engines. Technical improvements are needed before they become a good buy.

▶ Switch to lead-free petrol and think about having a catalytic converter installed.

▶ Slow down to save petrol. Consumption is highest in start-and-stop town traffic and over 55 m.p.h. on the motorway.

▶ Avoid slamming on the brakes, use gears to slow down and don't rev the engine. Aggressive driving uses 20 per cent more petrol.

▶ Keep your car in good repair, regularly tuned and tyres fully inflated. Use radial tyres.
▶ Fit an electronic ignition.
▶ Remove roof racks when not in use. Wind resistance means increased petrol consumption.
▶ Lighter loads make for better mileage, so empty out the boot.
▶ Use asbestos-free brake pads – ring accessory shops or ask your garage.

HOLIDAYS

The overwhelming importance we attach to holiday plans might be seen as a sign that many of us are not happy with life at home. Often holidays are disappointing. Think how many people you've seen come back from a holiday looking tired and stressed, with only a pile of photos, credit card bills and a few amusing stories to tell at the office.

Tourism can be seen as a sort of pollution, something which destroys the thing it loves. People talk about Mauritius or Acapulco 'before it was spoiled'. Hotel complexes line the seafront in popular mass market resorts, catering standards degenerate to ubiquitous fast food, and the real life of the region disappears. Added to this is the extremely serious effect tourism has on the ecology of many precious wilderness areas.

Tourism in the third world has heavy social and cultural prices, borne by local people. Unfortunately, the notion that tourism can bring jobs and prosperity to poor regions is not confirmed by recent studies, which have found that at least 80 per cent of the money spent on holidays in the third world comes back to home countries, in foreign staff salaries, foreign-owned hotel profits, travel agency commissions, payment for imported food, and other items, insurance and interest on loans. Most of the remaining 20 per cent goes to a few wealthy locals and government officials.

The tourist industry generates only unskilled jobs – responsible positions tend to go to foreign employees – while causing a disruption of local life. Customs and religious rituals are transformed into spectacles, and traditional crafts become souvenirs.

Next time you sit down with a pile of glossy holiday brochures it's worth taking stock of what you really want to get out of this trip, especially when you consider the costs. One of the main reasons we go on holiday is to have a break from routine, to recharge our batteries. A camping trip or walking holiday may sound strenuous and tiring, but can do more to energize you than two weeks at a crowded resort. Here are some things to think about while you plan next summer's trip.

▶ How will you travel? Walking and cycling are good for you, and put you in contact with the places you visit. They also give you fresh air, exercise and a leisurely pace.

▶ You may be able to travel by train instead of car. Cars can go on the train – getting you to the South of France quickly and pleasantly, though not especially cheaply – or you can hire one at the other end.

▶ Instead of 'doing' sights, or towns, or countries, choose a spot which holds some genuine interest and read up about it in advance. This will not only make your visit more rewarding but will help you to fit in while you are there.

▶ Avoid package tours to resorts, described as 'mobile ghettos' because they give the tourist no contact with anyone whose job is not servicing tourists.

▶ Instead of looking for a home-away-from-home, think of holidays as a chance to experience something different from your regular way of life. Options include Outward Bound, Earthwatch and Working Weekends (or longer) on Organic Farms (WWOOF). See Sources.

▶ Eco-tourism is a booming business. It may not save wilderness or preserve indigenous cultures, but it's a better option than other package holidays.

▶ Respect for other people's feelings and customs is the most important thing you can take with you, whether you stay in Britain or travel abroad.

▶ If you are concerned about the impact of tourism on other countries, contact one of the groups listed in Sources.

■ Greener Travel

▶ Use B&Bs and small owner-run hotels instead of chain hotels to put your money into the local economy.

▶ Don't over-use towels and hot water just because you're not paying extra for them.

▶ Stay at hotels that are switching to conscious green practices, such as limiting sheet and towel changes, and installing low-water showerheads (they, like other businesses, are conscious that green practices save money).

▶ Leave those little bottles of shampoo at the hotel; they waste packaging and you don't need them.

▶ When you travel by air, ring ahead and order vegetarian meals.

▶ There seems to be more wasteful packaging and disposable products on aeroplanes than anywhere else – turn down all the over-packaged extras and write to the airline asking for better environmental policies.

GETTING AROUND SIMPLIFIED

• Take care of all your errands at one time.

• Limit shopping to one day a week.

• Choose a simple, well-made car and keep it a long time.

• Buy a second-hand car with cash.

• Take the train and catch up on your reading.

• Work at home or live near where you work.

• Take a holiday at home – no packing!

• Slow down: don't overbook yourself and stop racing.

• Co-ordinate packages sent by courier and, if you use mail order, order in bulk.

• Use electronic mail and fax, rather than courier services.

• Ask for, or offer, interest-free loans for public transport season tickets.

9

THE AIR WE BREATHE

Our sense of smell is controlled by the primitive part of the brain, closely connected with the parts of the brain which control emotion, mood and personality, and it plays a key role in sexual attraction. Smell gave our ancestors information about the world and it can be a source of considerable pleasure. But smell has become a neglected sense. We get little information about a modern city environment through our noses. We tune out noxious smells because we have little control over them. Indoors, we smother ourselves in artificial fragrances.

Modern life bombards us with manufactured odours from the time we are born. Scented baby lotions, powders and even disposable nappies interfere with our olfactory awareness. But it is possible to create a home environment free of most of these artificial scents, and one's sense of smell and taste can recover their acuity (because our sense of taste depends on our ability to smell, dullness of one leads to dullness of the other).

Move to an open window or go outside. Close your eyes and take several long, deep breaths. Fill your lungs all the way down to your stomach. Can you remember times when breathing has been a conscious pleasure? Shallow, inadequate breathing is characteristic of sedentary people and perhaps our heedless pollution of the air around us has something to do with the fact that we don't get enough exercise to breathe with appreciation. One of the many benefits of getting fit is a clearer awareness of the environment.

AIR POLLUTION

The acrid, brown haze that lies over most large cities is largely the result of burning fossil fuels, and comes from car exhaust and industrial emissions. Urban air pollution is not new. London air was often black during the days of coal fires. Clean air legislation had dramatic effects after the Second World War – when a temperature inversion trapped the air over London for several days in 1952 and some 4000 people died – but air pollution remains a serious problem throughout the world, causing illness and death, the crumbling of historic buildings and monuments, and damage to trees and wildlife.

Air pollution damages the delicate linings of the nose, throat and lungs, causing a variety of respiratory complaints, while in the lungs it can enter the bloodstream and reach other parts of the body. Some of the chemicals in typical urban smog have been found to alter DNA in cells to cause cancer and birth defects. More subtly, it also suppresses the immune system by reducing lymphocyte and antibody production, making us more susceptible to illness.

TOXIC CLOUDS

While the contamination of water is a great problem, the speed with which toxic materials move through the air, carried by the winds, makes the pollution of air an increasing threat to human health and to the environment. The Aral Sea in south central Asia was the fourth largest inland sea until intensive irrigation of the surrounding region from the rivers which fed it caused its shores to recede dramatically. The salt left exposed is caught up in huge windstorms and deposited over an area of many thousands of miles, salinating the soil and making agriculture even more difficult.

Even the most remote areas are affected. In 1982 the US Environmental Protection Agency found high levels of toxaphene (a highly carcinogenic insecticide), PCBs, dioxins and DDT by-products in an isolated part of Lake Superior in the northern US. Toxaphene was never used in significant quantities by farmers in that part of the country, and researchers concluded that the poisons must have travelled by air from the cotton fields of the southern US, more than 1000 miles away.

'Toxic fallout' is made up of solid particles, invisible gases and aerosol mists, and it may be responsible for thousands of cancers and genetic mutations. Aside from the known hazards related to individual chemicals, there is the unpredictable danger of what those chemicals will do in combination or of what the cumulative effect will be as they build up in the atmosphere. Our experience so far with CFCs doesn't give a good prognosis.

You may think that severe air pollution is confined to large urban areas, but the fact is that some people have to move into the city in order to get away from agricultural chemicals. Looking at Britain's pastoral, patchwork landscape, this is a chilling thought. Modern agriculture is a source of some of the most dangerous chemicals in use because they are specifically designed to kill living organisms. Many do not break down in the environment. Country folk, from farm workers to weekending stockbrokers, face problems with nitrate fertilizers and agricultural chemicals in drinking water, and dangerous and debilitating contamination from aerial crop spraying.

In addition, many pesticides are applied by aerial spraying, which is inadequately regulated and monitored. Friends of the Earth has compiled a dossier of dozens of incidents of people being sprayed with poisonous chemicals. The most horrific was a case in which a group of schoolchildren were directly and repeatedly sprayed by an aircraft while they stood waving at it.

ACTION FOR CLEAN AIR

▶ Buy organically grown food (Chapter 5).
▶ Conserve energy (Chapter 7).
▶ Drive less and choose unleaded petrol (Chapter 8).
▶ Do not buy products containing CFCs (Chapter 3).
▶ Do not use aerosol products (this chapter).
▶ Use non-toxic domestic products (Chapter 12).
▶ Plant trees (Chapter 15).
▶ Write to your MP about the regulation of hazardous chemicals, including pesticides (see Postscript, page 290, for tips about writing letters).

■ Personal Checklist

▶ Spend as much time as possible outdoors, preferably in clean air spots (such as mountains, beaches and some parts of the countryside).
▶ Increase ventilation at home.
▶ Avoid synthetic materials.
▶ Stay away from smokers.
▶ Carry or wear a silk scarf to cover your mouth and nose in or near heavy traffic. Many cyclists wear special masks.

INDOOR AIR POLLUTION

A study by the US Environmental Protection Agency found that 'People are exposed to more potentially harmful pollutants indoors – at home, in the office, and in the car – than outdoors. . . . The worst household dangers identified so far include smoking, living with a smoker, using air fresheners, moth crystals, aerosol sprays and storing paints and solvents.'

Tobacco smoke is by far the worst kind of indoor air pollution, with proven health risks for non-smokers and especially for children, but many other common products pollute the air we breathe. Heaters and cookers use up fresh air and give off vapours, so good ventilation is essential if you use gas appliances or paraffin heaters (have your appliances serviced regularly, too). And solvents – found in art supplies, glues, varnishes, paints and other household products – can be particularly hazardous.

Our increasingly energy-efficient houses are leading to more air pollution because concentration of gases from building materials and domestic products are allowed to build up to dangerous levels, and we spend an increasing amount of time indoors. Better draughtproofing has been linked to increased asthma in children, not because there is anything wrong with draughtproofing, but because it means that we spend much of our time in a bell jar full of hazardous chemicals. Removing indoor toxins should go hand in hand with energy conservation.

US army doctors at the Walter Reed Army Institute found that colds and flu are less likely in draughty buildings. They attributed this to a build-up of viruses in well-sealed buildings, but it may be that fresh air is needed to keep our immune systems functioning effectively. Many people find themselves suffering from regular colds as soon as the central heating is turned on (and the windows are closed) in the autumn. The dry, stuffy atmosphere of centrally heated buildings affects our respiratory systems and makes us more vulnerable to whatever viruses are about.

HAZARDOUS PRODUCTS

Cleaning up the air inside your home is a matter of making some changes in the cleaning products you use, allowing new carpets and furniture to 'out-gas' vapours, or choosing untreated floor coverings and furniture made from natural, untreated materials. This subject is covered at length in Chapter 12 (see also p. 95), but here are a few points specifically related to air pollution.

Cleaning products can be hazardous and warnings on packages do not always mention the hazards of breathing the volatile fumes given off by many products. If chlorine bleach and ammonia, both extremely common household cleaners, are mixed they produce a gas which can cause death within minutes. You can make your own inexpensive cleaning products, or buy a number of commercial products which are safe for you, for children and pets, and for the environment.

Toiletries, such as the acetone in nail polish remover, can pollute inside air. The same is true of the harsh synthetic fragrances in many cosmetics and shampoos.

Aerosols, whether CFC-based or not, are a source of indoor air pollution. Because they disperse their contents as an extremely fine mist, products which contain toxic ingredients (such as hairspray and insecticide) can be inhaled and easily enter the bloodstream. Certain propellant gases are themselves lung irritants and depress the central nervous system. Medical specialists including the American Lung Association advise against their use. You can always find a non-aerosol equivalent: pump action, liquid or cream products work very well.

Commercial air fresheners are potentially dangerous and certainly unnecessary. Some brands simply disguise bad smells with another strong scent, while others work by coating nasal passages with a fine oil film or by releasing a chemical which deadens your olfactory nerves. When you want to add a pleasant scent to the air, or to disguise an unpleasant smell, use one of the natural air fresheners suggested below, p. 153.

DIY, HOBBY AND OFFICE PRODUCTS

Many of these contain hydrocarbon solvents, which are so toxic that they can cause death by inhalation. Take great care when using them, use as little as possible and choose alternative products when you can.

Your nose is a good guide. As adhesives dry, they out-gas various chemicals. Sealants which stay soft will continue to do so for years. Even paint can cause problems for sensitive people – stay away from new paint or varnish until the smell has disappeared, or at least keep windows open. In any case, circulating air speeds drying more effectively than heat.

In general, choose materials that are hard or dry hard (brittle rather than soft plastic, for example) and which have no perceptible smell. See Chapter 12 for more information.

PESTICIDES

Avoiding chemical insecticides is crucial inside your home. Indoor plants can be raised organically (see Chapter 15). Organic pest control methods are safe but they may not smell wonderful, so move the plants you are treating outside.

See Chapter 12, pp. 197–9 for non-toxic methods of dealing with household pests such as flies and moths.

HEATING AND HUMIDITY

Electrical appliances give out no fumes, but they are less effective as a source of domestic energy than gas appliances and there is considerable scientific concern about the effects of living with high levels of electromagnetic radiation.

In a draughtproofed house it is especially important to see that gas and wood fires are properly vented. Gas ranges should burn with a blue flame – if yours has orange flames ask the gas board to come and adjust it – and the kitchen needs a vent or fan to remove combustion by-products. Many health specialists advise against the use of any unvented gas or paraffin heater. If you use this form of heat, ensure that there is plenty of ventilation.

Central heating creates a dry atmosphere – some people have trouble with sore throats when the central heating is switched on, and the low humidity is hard on plants and furniture. One solution to this problem is a humidifier, but acquiring an energy-hungry appliance to counteract the effects of an unsatisfactory method of heating seems silly. Humidifiers can also have the bacterial growth found in air-conditioning systems. Combination heating is probably the best solution: using radiant heat sources whenever possible and saving the central heating for very cold weather. A well-insulated house doesn't need a great deal of heating in milder weather, especially if there is a considerable amount of thermal inertia.

Humidity can be increased by keeping bowls of water around (the speed at which they evaporate will give you a clue as to just how dry your home gets) and by having plenty of plants inside (plants suffer as least as much as we do from central heating, but can be arranged in such a way as to add moisture to the air).

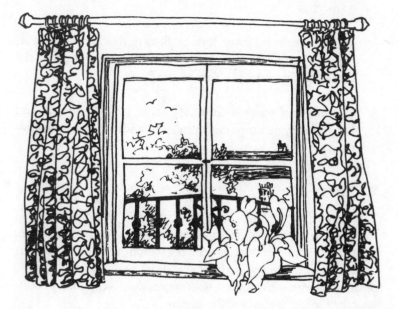

IMPROVING THE AIR

To improve the air you breathe at home, in the summer you can throw the windows open, but during the colder months the following ideas are especially important.

1. Declare your home a non-smoking zone. If you don't feel you can go quite that far, establish that smokers can only use a particular room, which can be aired easily. Or ask that smokers step outside with their cigarettes.

2. Research into 'sick office syndrome' has found that still air 'feels' stuffy – you need air movement, while avoiding direct draughts.

3. According to the *National Trust Manual of Housekeeping*, still air, like still water, encourages bacterial growth. Open strategic windows for a daily airing. Various essential oils, including lavender and tea tree, are said to have antibacterial properties.

4. Don't overheat your home. Steady background heat, together with specific sources of radiant heat, may be the best solution to the problem of stuffiness.

5. Use bowls of water to humidify the air. If you do this, and keep the temperature moderate, a humidifier will be unnecessary.

■Ionizers

Air-conditioning and heating systems, cigarette smoke, electronic equipment of all kinds and synthetic carpeting change the balance of ions in the air. Air near running water is refreshing and invigorating in part because of its negative ion charge; a positive charge is associated with increased susceptibility to illness, including hayfever and migraine.

Using fewer electrical appliances and more natural materials in your home, along with good ventilation, may solve part of the problem, but an ionizer, which creates a negative charge in the air, makes a perceptible improvement in the indoor environment for many people. Ionizers are relatively inexpensive and use very little power.

In offices, they have been found to increase alertness and productivity. People who spend a great deal of time in front of a visual display unit (VDU) screen are exposed to some 50 times the positive ion charge of someone who does not use a VDU. The screen repels positively charged particles on to the face and into the lungs of the user – a likely reason for the increase in bronchial and skin disorders, and conjunctivitis among VDU operators.

If you use an ionizer, point it at you, as the effect is directional. Turn it off during the day if you use it at night or vice versa – the change in ion concentration is important for the metabolism.

■Plants

Plants improve the environment. They increase the oxygen content of the air, act as a humidifier and can even filter the air to some degree. Plants and vases of flowers give off water and oxygen, so both will improve the air – and fragrant flowers or foliage will add their scent too. The common spider plant (*Chlorophytum*) and golden pothos (*Scindapsus aureus*) are said to reduce indoor toxins, but all plants will improve the quality of the air you breathe. Spider plants actually remove formaldehyde, a common irritant in modern buildings, from the air.

Plants stay healthier if they are grouped together. This increases the humidity of the air around them, and an easy way to see that their atmosphere stays moist as well as increasing the general level of humidity is to stand them on trays of pebbles which you keep topped up with water. The plant pots should not be in the water – many plants will die if their roots are waterlogged – but just clear of it.

■Natural Air Fresheners

The best freshener, of course, is fresh air. But throughout history people have used the scents of herbs and flowers to enhance the atmosphere in a room as well as to disguise unpleasant odours.

Pot-pourri means 'rotten pot', because they were originally fermented mixtures of flowers and herbs. The pot-pourri many of us are familiar with is a dry blend based on rose petals and lavender. These look pretty but do not usually have a strong aroma. An occasional stirring releases the fragrance, and adding extra essential oils from time to time will increase their effectiveness. Blends vary, and you can make your own with garden flowers or purchased ingredients.

More potent mixtures are fermented with salt, and need to be kept in covered pot-pourri jars – they smell delightful but are not so attractive. Pot-pourris do not have to be flowery. A mixture based on spices – cinnamon, cloves, vanilla pods – is an intriguing alternative.

Fill a dish, and your car's ashtray, with a mixture of whole cloves and cinnamon bark. (It's cheapest to buy spices in bulk at a wholefood store, and they last for ages). A quick shake raises the scent. Another fast trick, which smells delightful and is useful if you've just burned something in the kitchen, is to boil a few pieces of orange or lemon rind in a small saucepan of water. Cinnamon and cloves work equally well.

Even easier to use are essential oils distilled from plants and flowers. You'll find these little bottles of scent remarkably useful around the house. (A word of warning, however – be careful about what you buy. Some 'aromatherapy' oils are diluted in soyabean oil, making them quite expensive compared with pure essential oils, which you can dilute yourself.) They are quite essential in the green home, added to home-made cleaning products or a simple vinegar hair rinse. You can put 10–20 drops of pine or rosemary oil into a bath with a handful of sea salt. A few drops of cinnamon oil on a lightbulb will make it smell as if you've been baking or you can rub a few drops of lavender oil into your temples when you are feeling tired. If you can go to a shop which sells essential oils, you can sniff test several dozen and start a collection.

The oils can also be used in small pottery burners – the natural alternative to chemical air fresheners. Some scents – ginger and patchouli for example – are said to have aphrodisiacal properties, so keep those in the bedroom!

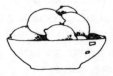

10

WATER

Our major cities were built beside water, and as human societies have developed, their interactions with the natural
water supply become more and more complex. Water is pumped
from rivers and aquifers to provide running water in homes and
factories, to generate energy, to irrigate fields. Valleys are flooded
to store water for large cities and hydro-electric dams. Along the
Mississippi, in the central US, towns that have existed for over a
century stand in floodplains, with the river held back by a system
of levies.

While rivers, lakes and oceans have been dumping grounds for
millennia, when the world's population was smaller and the
waste less toxic, the water – full of animals, plants and bacteria –
was able to render it harmless. Modern waste, however, is not
only non-degradable but highly toxic, and the natural cycles of
lakes and rivers cannot clean it up.

Water is a potent symbol in our culture. Our earth is the water
planet, with some 75 per cent of its surface covered by water, and
human beings are made largely of water too, as any schoolchild
can explain. Life throughout the centuries has been tied to the
natural rhythms of rivers, bays and coastlines. But over the past

century or so, natural sources of water have been covered over and lost to us, in order to fit the exigencies of 'rational' town planning. In London, dozens of smaller rivers have been routed underground (the Fleet gave its name to Fleet Street), indoor swimming pools are heavily chlorinated and lit by fluorescent lights, and even the ponds in parks are often fenced off.

This is a pity. We need contact with water. There are few things more pleasant and soothing than the sound of running water. Natural streams could be maintained and preserved, for our use and to encourage wildlife. Appreciative attitudes towards, and a sense of connection with, the water around us is a vital step in stopping our pollution of it.

WATER POLLUTION

Industrial chemicals, toxic materials of all sorts, oil and even nuclear waste are ignominiously dumped into our streams and rivers, and the sea. Many beaches would be shut down as unsafe if they were in another country: according to Greenpeace, 'tests [in Blackpool] have shown a concentration of bacteria and viruses from sewage in the sea-water 50 times above the safety limits set by Canadian public health authorities'.

Raw, untreated sewage is sometimes piped straight from sewers into the sea close to bathing beaches. Even worse, UK regulations allow toxic industrial wastes to be discharged into the same sewers as domestic sewage (which could be processed as a valuable fertilizer). Contaminated sewage sludge, containing cadmium and mercury, lindane and DDT, has been associated with the deaths of seabirds in the Thames estuary and Greenpeace says that London sewage is a likely contributor to the deaths of thousands of seals in the North Sea.

We all contribute to the pollution of the earth's water and our own water supplies, and need to understand the connection between what we pour down the drain or flush down the toilet and reports of animal deaths on the news. Rachel Carson wrote in 1962 that 'In the entire water-pollution problem there is prob-

ably nothing more disturbing than the threat of widespread contamination of groundwater. It is not possible to add pesticides to
water anywhere without threatening the purity of water everywhere.'

In many areas, people can tell that there is something wrong
with their water by the fact that it smells and tastes so bad. But
most of the 700 or so known chemical contaminants in public
drinking water are not detectable to the nose or eye or taste. Just
because your water looks all right doesn't mean that it is good for
you. The following is a summary of the major problems facing
our water supplies.

■Fertilizers

Nitrate fertilizers pose a serious threat to water supplies. More
than 3 million tonnes are used in the UK every year. Of this,
approximately half is taken up by the crops and the remainder is
washed out of the soil, into our water. In rivers and lakes nitrates
contribute to excessive algae growth, which tends to choke other
plant and animal life. The nitrates slowly seep into deep boreholes and formerly pure groundwater. Even now a third of
British water supplies contain higher nitrate levels than the EC
maximum recommended limit.

The nitrates in the water we are drinking now were probably
applied to the land 20–40 years ago. Since nitrate use has been
much heavier since the 1960s, we can only expect the problem of
nitrate contamination to become worse.

In the body, nitrates are reduced to nitrites and nitrosamines,
which have been strongly implicated in stomach and oesophageal
cancer. They are especially dangerous for babies because they are
thought to cause the potentially fatal 'blue baby syndrome'. In
spite of this, the government has fought the EC regulations and
is only slowly facing the long-term health threat posed by
nitrates.

■Pesticides

Water containing a high level of nitrates is almost certain to contain agricultural pesticides as well. If you consider the tonnes of toxic chemicals used each year to kill insects and weeds, it is not surprising that a substantial amount should reach us via our water supplies. The link between agricultural pollution from organophosphate pesticides, and various hormonal changes and health problems in humans, as well as in fish and animal life, is discussed in Chapter 5. A switch to organic farming methods will cut pesticide use and in the mean time we can have little choice but to drink whatever happens to be in our tap water. Some filtration systems, however, will remove a high percentage of pesticides from drinking water (see below, pp. 166–7).

■Slurry And Sewage

Modern large-scale farming is done on a single crop basis: pigs or wheat or rape or potatoes. This does not lend itself to the ecological farming practices of a traditional mixed farm, where animals grazed on rough grass, ate plant stalks and, naturally, provided fertilizer for the next year's crop. Intensively reared, factory-farmed animals – pigs and cattle, as well as chickens – produce manure, but it is treated as a disposal problem instead of as a rich source of fertilizer. The waste slurry contaminates water supplies. Routinely administered antibiotics, used as growth promoters, also enter the soil and water in this way.

In the past, human waste was garnered by farmers as carefully as animal waste. The soil produced food, and everything was returned to it in a beneficial and sustainable system. But as people have moved into cities, it has become a disposal problem instead of a recycling material.

It's not a pleasant thought, but much of the water we drink has been reprocessed from effluent, the water and sewage we use and send down the drain. All our water, not just the water we drink or bathe in, is expensively purified, and questionable chemicals are added to it in the process.

In towns and cities there is not much alternative to a centralized system, but this could be designed to make use of waste rather than treat it as a nuisance. One advantage of a centralized system is that sewage can also be used to produce energy in the form of methane gas. There are a number of programmes in development that use plants and/or natural biological processes to speed the breaking down of sewage.

Composting at source is another good choice because it does without pipes and tanks and transport. Anyone with land can use one of the modern composting systems (instead of a septic tank, if that's what you have now) which use both kitchen/household scraps and toilet waste to make a rich, safe fertilizer. You may feel squeamish about this, but then you probably don't want to know just where the water which went into your tea this morning came from! The Centre for Alternative Technology in Powys can provide information (see Sources, p. 300).

■Detergents

Synthetic detergents are types of soap developed during the rise of the petrochemical industry, notable for being effective in both hard and soft water. They are in common use, in household cleaning supplies, in industrial cleaning, dyeing and bleaching, and in making cosmetics. Household detergents contain softeners, bleaches, brighteners and enzymes, and most contain phosphates.

Eutrophication is one of the results of our excessive use of synthetic detergents. It means 'to become rich in food' and leads to a rapid ageing of lakes and streams as plant life grows far more rapidly than it would under normal conditions. When the water in a lake, river wetland or even in coastal areas becomes too rich in phosphates from detergents and nitrates from fertilizers there is excessive growth of algae. Other forms of water life, including fish, die.

Switzerland has banned phosphates because of concern about their lakes and other countries should follow suit. Switch to biodegradable, phosphate-free cleaning products. You can make your own, and there are several excellent commercial ranges available.

■Chlorine

The most obvious characteristic of modern tap water is the smell of chlorine, which is unpleasant at best. Some people have allergic reactions to it. Far worse, chlorine combines with the natural acids in water from peaty soil and decomposing vegetable matter (leaves, for example) to form chloroform, a toxic compound. It has been known for some years that there are significantly higher death rates from gastrointestinal and urinary tract cancers among people drinking chlorinated water.

■Aluminium

Aluminium sulphate is added in huge quantities (100,000 tonnes a year, at a cost of £7 million) to UK water supplies, to settle out solid impurities such as dissolved peat. Acid rain caused by pollution has increased the amount of aluminium in our water too, because it dissolves the otherwise inert and harmless aluminium found in certain soils. Aluminium is implicated in senile dementia and Alzheimer's disease, and experts recommend that we all cut down on the amount we ingest. Its effect is cumulative and long term, unlike lead which affects brain development in a relatively short period of time.

■Plumbing

Most people know that lead water pipes were common in homes built before 1900 and many of these pipes have been replaced. But what many of us are unaware of is that the joints in our new copper pipes are sealed with lead solder (as are tin cans) and these too are a source of lead. A Water Research Council report advised against the use of lead solder for pipes carrying drinking water. At present, the alternatives are mechanical rather than soldered fittings, or a special 95/5 solder (made for heating systems) which contains only a tenth as much lead as the standard 50/50 solder.

The leaching of lead into water is accelerated by the presence of chlorine and other chemicals, soft water will dissolve more heavy metals than hard water, and hot water more than cold.

■Toxic Chemicals

The waste from manufacturing products is often disposed of by pumping it into the nearest river or ocean. Major aquifers are now contaminated by effluents from industrial waste, and these problems have led to legislation about dumping and landfill in some industrialized countries, and precipitated the new international market in domestic and industrial waste.

Waste disposal is a growing problem and solid waste disposal sites are one of the biggest sources of groundwater contamination. Military sites are among the most contaminated places on earth, and as they are closed in the post Cold War peace, governments are looking for ways to clean up the sites, and neighbouring towns too.

Toxic chemicals get into our water in other ways, too. Accidental spills of sulphuric acid and other chemicals wreak havoc on water life. Oil spills at sea are common, and it is thought that some 5 tons of highly toxic PCBs were released into the North Sea when the Piper Alpha oil platform exploded in 1988. Leakage from underground petrol storage tanks is not uncommon.

■Drugs

The drugs we consume are eventually excreted and flushed away, and we are often advised to dispose of unused drugs by dumping them down the loo to prevent their getting into the hands of children. Drugs do not necessarily biodegrade, but biodegradability is not a determining factor for the pharmaceutical industry. We need to keep in mind that drugs are synthetic chemicals, many produced by the world's largest chemical firms, and some of them enter our water supplies. It is better to return any unused drugs to the doctor.

There have been questions raised about cytotoxic cancer drugs, thought to be particularly hazardous. The Women's Environmental Network is concerned about water supplies being polluted with oestrogen, a human hormone, from birth control pills. Of course the amounts are minute, but the quantity of chemicals or drugs posing a risk to human health depends a great deal on individual tolerances, and studies of risk differ greatly. And we don't know about the effects of even minute quantities of hazardous drugs in combination.

This would seem to be a good reason to cut drastically our dependence on drugs, and to use more complementary medicine and homeopathy.

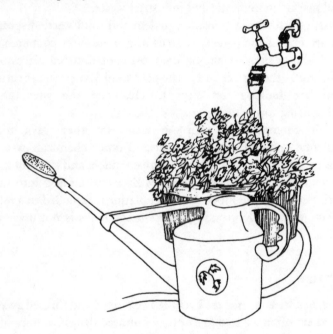

WATER CONSERVATION

Conserving water in Britain seems crazy, most of the time. When I hang clothes outdoors to dry, even in summer, it can be a performance trying to get everything dry between cloudbursts. I've had clothes hanging outside for days, alternately wet and dry on a schedule that never quite coincided with mine. But we do have droughts, because of changing weather patterns, and increased population and water use in certain regions. So much ground-water is used in and around urban areas that the 'water table', the normal depth of the sub-surface groundwater, is sinking.

We have affected the earth's natural water cycles as the demand for water increases. Lavatories, washing machines, dish-washers, swimming pools, irrigation, industrial cleaning and cooling are some of the ways we use water from rivers, reservoirs and from deep underground aquifers. Valleys are flooded, and villages and woods are lost in order to make reservoirs to supply drinking water for us. The lowering of the water table is a prob-lem even in Britain and a serious one in many other parts of the world.

In any case, we shouldn't equate the water that pours from the sky with the water we need to conserve, which comes from the tap. The former is an abundant natural resource, whereas the lat-ter has undergone considerable processing, with a wide range of ecological and environmental consequences. Water metering could have positive effects, if it helped us to be more careful with the water we use. Unfortunately, the near doubling of water bills since privatization in 1989 does not seem to have led to improve-ments in either the quality of our water or our environment.

The real lunacy of our present system is that our drinking water is not clean enough to drink with complete confidence, while the water we use for other purposes, bathing and washing clothes and watering the garden, is cleaner than it need be. In the future, we need more complex domestic plumbing in order to use water efficiently. In *Blueprint for a Green Planet*, John Seymour and Herbert Giradet suggested that the present one pipe system should be replaced with a dual water system. Drinking and wash-ing water would come from underground boreholes and springs, and would not need the addition of chlorine. It would taste good! All other water, for industrial use, watering the garden, washing the car and flushing the loo, would get a minimal filtering.

This might not be as expensive as it sounds because many British water systems are due for renewal and in any case you could certainly adapt your own household's plumbing with some help from the Centre for Alternative Technology or the EDA (see Sources, p. 300). A variation on the theme is the use of 'grey water' systems for low grade uses, particularly in gardens. Household water is used twice, first for cooking and washing (with biodegradable and non-toxic soaps), then for watering the garden.

WATER CHECKLIST

- Don't waste water: turn off the tap while you brush your teeth, shave or condition your hair.
- Stop leaks.
- Have showers instead of baths.
- Install a low-flow shower head.
- Run the washing machine with a full load. Front-opening washing machines are more efficient than top-loading machines, using less energy and less water. (More efficient washing machines coming on to the market have a suds-saver feature, saving rinse water for the next wash cycle.)
- Install an instant water heater, doing away with the tank (this saves energy too).
- Insulate hot water pipes so you don't need to let water run for long.
- Run full loads in the dishwasher. Scrape dishes instead of rinsing before putting into the dishwasher.
- Do the washing up in a small bowl of very hot water, and rinse everything at once.
- Wash vegetables in a small bowl of water, rather than under the tap.
- Use the light wash cycle.
- Save rainwater and use in the garden, or to wash the car or bicycle.
- Choose plants which don't need to be water frequently.
- Mulch garden beds.
- Water with a drop hose early in the morning or in the evening.

- Low flush loos are becoming common in arid parts of the US and can be installed in Britain.
- Adapt the loo to take less water on each flush (see illustration below).
- Many old-fashioned water closets, with suspended tanks of water, use less water than modern flush lavatories. They are more noisy but if you have one that does its job, keep it as an example of water-conserving technology.

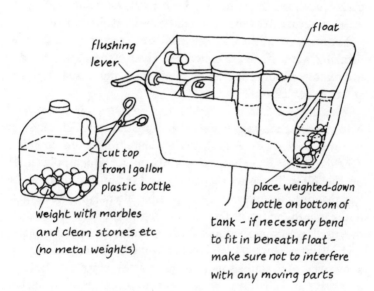

float

flushing lever

cut top from 1 gallon plastic bottle

weight with marbles and clean stones etc (no metal weights)

place weighted-down bottle on bottom of tank - if necessary bend to fit in beneath float - make sure not to interfere with any moving parts

Ecological water cistern

DRINKING WATER

Anyone on a diet will know that the standard advice is to drink lots of water because it fills you up and flushes you out. Eight glasses a day is a suggested target for good health. Water is good for our systems, and skin is moister and clearer when you have plenty of it to drink.

If you use ordinary tap water, run cold water for cooking and drinking, and flush the pipes with cold water for several minutes first thing in the morning.

Bottled waters may be pleasant but they are bad news for the environment. Processing, packaging and transporting water around the world is wasteful and should not be necessary. If you drink bottled water for flavour or because you're afraid to drink water from the tap, buy the largest bottles you can of the water that comes from closest to home. This will minimize the ecological costs. Choose glass bottles if you can. Water bottled in plastic absorbs a certain quantity of possibly carcinogenic polymers and glass bottles are easier to recycle. A local source of fresh spring water in returnable bottles would be an ideal alternative.

For many of us, there is little choice at present but to filter our drinking water if we are concerned about its quality. This does not remove all impurities, but gives a safer, more palatable drink at a reasonable price.

There are a number of filtration systems on the market. Effectiveness, and the chemicals and pollutants which each type removes, varies a great deal. Prices range from a few pounds to £500 or more. The cheapest is a plastic jug which holds a disposable filter. These are easy to use and reasonably effective, but less than ideal because of the disposable filters (you need at least one a month, and probably more often as they are dangerous if overused, releasing the filtered heavy metals and possibly bacteria back into the water). A glass jug would be better, and there are a number of plumbed-in systems on the market. These are expensive initially but work out considerably cheaper in the long run and have fewer disposable parts.

There are three basic methods of filtration and the appropriate type depends on your water supply.

1. **Activated carbon** is inexpensive and removes chlorine, pesticides and organic chemicals, but not fluoride or nitrates. A carbon block filter may also remove heavy metals. Choose a granulated rather than powdered carbon filter as it is less prone to bacterial growth.

2. **Reverse osmosis (R/O)** uses a fine cellulose or plastic membrane to filter water under pressure, and removes asbestos, bacteria and viruses, fluoride, aluminium, heavy metals, minerals, salts and nitrates. R/O removes all minerals, even desirable ones like calcium and magnesium (which contribute to the pleasant taste of a good mineral water), and the output water is said to be very acid.

3. **Distillation** is promoted as being 'closest to nature' because rainwater, too, is distilled. The natural water we would drink by choice, however, is spring water, which is filtered through many layers of rock, absorbing valuable minerals and flavour. Distilled water is pure but insipid, requires a great deal of energy to produce (6p worth of electricity per litre) and is slow. On the other hand, distillation is extremely effective at removing contaminants, although care has to be taken to ensure that volatile organic chemicals are not condensed along with the steam.

The purest water comes either from a distiller or from a reverse osmosis unit used in conjunction with a carbon pre-filter. You should get an analysis of your local water supply from the water authority before deciding on a system and insist on having laboratory test results from any supplier (especially if you are buying one of the more expensive systems). Enquire about how best to avoid bacterial growth in the filter – the most important thing is to change the cartridge as directed. As public concern about our water supply increases, unscrupulous manufacturers are bound to get into the filter market. They can easily make unsubstantiated claims, especially as there are no British Standards for this product yet.

Some water authorities discourage the use of home water filters, claiming they are dangerous because of the possibility of bacterial growth, and insisting that the standard of public water supplies in England and Wales is high and becoming higher, although they admit nitrates are a growing problem which requires government action.

HEALING WATER

The simplest water therapy is swimming – preferably in the open air in unchlorinated ocean or lake water. Swimming is the exercise or sport invariably suggested for people who are unfit, overweight, have bad backs or are pregnant, because it gives great health benefits without putting strain on the body.

On the continent, various water therapies have been popular for many years and there is a growing interest in Britain in cold water treatments. One called thermo-regulatory hydrotherapy (TRHT) is vaunted as a cure for chronic fatigue syndrome and other disorders. This is really an old-fashioned idea, using cold water as a way to stimulate the body's immune system and can be used at home. You might try cold showers or baths (followed by a rubdown and warm clothes), or outdoor swimming all year round.

While you can save water and energy by having a shower instead of a bath, bathing has a place in our lives, too. Consider the bath a sensual experience and ideally one to be shared. In Japan, the bathing room is a social centre. You wash in a small bucket of water, and get into a large communal bath of hot water to soak and relax. Some architects have taken this approach in planning bathing rooms as part of an ecological home, with insulated tubs and solar water heaters to reduce energy consumption, biodegradable soaps and shampoo, and a system for using bath water in the garden.

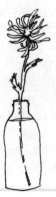

$\boxed{11}$

HEALTH
AND HEALING

Many people find that taking responsibility for their own health and health care leads them into greater concern for the environment. This is because our health provides a guide to the state of the environment we live in and because taking charge, studying and observing physical details and interconnections, becoming involved, gives one the confidence to question authority and demand satisfactory answers.

Human beings evolved over millennia to live in a certain physical and social environment. Physically, we are hunter–gatherers and the rapid technological changes of the past century have put our bodies in a vulnerable position because we are not adapted to the modern environment.

Allergies and food sensitivities are on the increase, heart disease and cancer are the so-called diseases of civilization, and most of us suffer from minor complaints which interfere to a greater or lesser degree with what we would like to do in our lives. Unfortunately, the assumption is that if something – say, petro-chemical products or chlorine in tap water – doesn't make us overtly ill, it must be OK. The subtle effects of low level radiation are ignored.

Our lives are cushioned, cocooned and sheltered in a way which our ancestors would not have been able to imagine. Fewer children die in infancy as a result, but as we grow up we lose out in becoming alienated from our bodies, as intrepid traveller Dervla Murphy reflects in her *In Ethiopia with a Mule* '. . . the machine-age has dangerously deprived Western man of whole areas of experience that until recently were common to the entire human race. Too many of us are now cut off from the basic sensual gratifications of resting after violent exercise, finding relief from extremes of heat or cold, eating when ravenously hungry and drinking when the ache of thirst makes water seem the most precious of God's creations.'

Although it is often difficult to connect specific aspects of the way we live with a particular health problem, there are many aspects of modern life which affect our state of health. The amount of time we spend indoors under artificial lighting in sealed buildings, uncomfortable seating, a long and stressful journey to work, electrical wiring and appliances, soulless architecture and traffic noise all affect the way we feel. Social factors such as crowding and crime are important too. People are put under stress and their health suffers when they no longer have safe public space, when they are on the defensive as soon as they step outside.

ATTITUDES TOWARDS HEALTH

The availability of medical attention and the overwhelming demands of modern life mean that many people abdicate all responsibility for their own health, and indeed become career patients. They want access to medication and high-tech medical care in emergencies, and ignore the other indignities that come with health problems – the irritating morning cough and breathlessness after climbing a few flights of stairs, for example, which plague many smokers. If you go for a physical examination – perhaps for a new job – and get a clean bill of health, you may still have bad breath, flat feet and frequent indigestion. Health has come to mean merely the absence of an obviously debilitating disease.

Do you get pleasure out of complaining about your aches and pains, about how you are working long hours, smoking too much, not getting enough exercise? Some people don't use a bicycle because they are embarrassed about going out on one, afraid they'll look awkward or silly, or because they worry about what people will think.

Illness has become something to conquer (advertisements for aspirin talk about 'hitting back at pain') with an instant remedy, so it doesn't interfere with our busy lives. We treat the body as a machine, which needs an occasional oiling and maybe a replacement part now and then, instead of as a complex and self-sustaining system.

An entirely different approach, taken by most alternative practitioners, is that illness is a positive thing because it tells us something is wrong. Fatigue is a sign that your body (and maybe your mind) needs a rest. Indigestion is a request for a change of diet. A chronically stiff neck might tell you that you are tense or that you're spending too much time hunched over your desk. Clinical ecologists point out that disease (eczema, for example) is not the primary event, but look to the cause (perhaps a sensitivity to milk) and try to treat that. The connection between the mind and body cannot be underestimated either. Continual colds may mean that you aren't eating well and your immune system isn't working well as a result, but they may also be a way avoiding a job you don't like, a way of asking for sympathy and support from those around you.

DEPENDENCE ON DRUGS

The pharmaceutical industry and the medical profession have disturbingly close links. Magazines aimed at general practitioners (GPs) have pages and pages of advertisements for pharmaceutical products, and all drug companies have reps who try to convince doctors to use their brands.

Some £3.2 billion is spent on drugs every year (£70,000 per GP) – 12.5 per cent of the NHS budget. The percentage is gradually rising. Britons are taking five times more prescription drugs than they were when the NHS was established in 1949. Are we five times as healthy when Britain has one of the highest rates of heart disease in the world?

Sadly, many doctors are far too busy to get to know patients, and often resort to prescribing drugs. How many women feel really free to ask about small worries when they find out they are pregnant? If a man comes in with a bad back, pain relief and bed rest are standard treatment. The fact that he is unemployed and having problems with his teenage children may not be taken into account.

Our attitudes towards doctors are at fault too, because many of us want an instant cure – we don't want to make changes in our lives and simply want some help in the process of compensation for ill health. Doctors sometimes claim that patients demand a prescription and they may write one on the assumption that taking something – or anything – will make the patient feel better. Even alternative remedies can be used irresponsibly because of our desire for instant relief without responsibility. I have seen the mothers of young children handing out tiny homeopathic pills for everything from whinging ('he must be teething') to a bruised knee ('arnica for shock'). A potent lesson is being conveyed. Vitamin pills can be used irresponsibly, too, and substituted for positive changes in the way we eat.

■ Antibiotics

Many serious infectious diseases, long thought to be under control, have in recent years re-emerged as significant health risks, and some experts believe that they pose a terrible threat to our society. These diseases – tuberculosis, rheumatic fever, meningitis and osteomyelitis – are emerging in mutant strains, resistant to known antibiotics. Hospitals have faced mini-plagues of bacteria which spread between patients via practitioners. The abuse of antibiotics, over-prescribed by doctors and overused or improperly taken by patients, is thought to be the cause. We also ingest antibiotics in animal products, because livestock is commonly dosed with antibiotics as a routine prophylactic and as growth promoters.

The problem of antibiotic abuse is even more serious in third world nations where trays of colourful antibiotic capsules – chloramphenicol, tetracycline or penicillin – are sold in street markets and hustled at train stations for everything from impotence to piles. Increased global travel connects us with antibiotic resistance developing among people in other parts of the world.

■Practical Measures On Medicine

Jeffrey A. Fisher, author of the *Plague Makers*, urges the following practices for doctors:

▶ fastidious handwashing, even when latex gloves are used;
▶ caution about prescribing antibiotics;
▶ testing of samples before prescription to ensure that the appropriate drug is used;
▶ use vaccination for elderly and other vulnerable patients in order to prevent flu which can lead to infection.

Patients should:

▶ instead of demanding inappropriate drugs, ask for guidelines on how to live healthily;
▶ if you do take an antibiotic, be sure to take it as prescribed and finish the full dose (this safeguards your own immune system and makes it less likely that mutant bacteria will grow in your system to pose a possible risk to other people);
▶ campaign for caution in the use of antibiotics and for legislation to end their use as growth promoters.

ALLERGIES

Allergies are an over-reaction of the immune system, the body's defence mechanisms, to irritating stimuli that the human body generally copes with without symptoms. The rise in allergies such as asthma, eczema and hayfever has had considerable press coverage, and it seems that few people do not consider themselves allergic to some food or household substance. This is not surprising when one considers the rapid increase in the number of new chemicals that have come into use in recent decades (see

Chapter 12). But allergic reactions are also connected with individual immune responses and we seem to be getting more sensitive to natural substances – pollen, for example – as well. Research suggests several causes for this increase.

First, we are able to provide far more hygienic surroundings than at any time in the past, so babies never develop strong immune systems. First-born children are more likely to suffer from allergies than other offspring and this may be because their early lives were more sheltered.

Second, only 25 per cent of British children are breastfed for the recommended minimum of four months. Breastfeeding is an important part of the process of developing strong immune systems, as a child is able to build its own immune system with help from its mother's antibodies. This is one reason breastfed babies are substantially healthier as infants and generally healthier throughout their lives.

Third, the pollution in our environment and the number of human-made chemical products we are exposed to in our homes and workplaces create an extra source of stress for weakened immune systems. A growing speciality called clinical ecology or environmental medicine concentrates on the way foods and food additives, chemicals, radiation and other pollutants cause disease, allergies, depression and fatigue.

ADAPTATION AND IMMUNITY

Good health means having the physical and psychological resources to respond to the demands of your life and environment. We don't get ill simply because there are viruses around. Bacteria, viruses, fungi and protozoa are with us all the time; we need many of them. Bacteria in our digestive tract help to digest food and organisms on our skin protect us from potentially harmful bacteria.

Illness often coincides with special pressure at work or coming back from holiday, or a diet of hamburgers and cola. The plight of seals in the North Sea has had important lessons for human beings. Like us, seals eat at the top of the food chain, and industrial pollutants like PCBs concentrate in their body fat. The poisons are released when they are under particular stress, when breeding and giving birth for example, depressing their immune systems making them vulnerable to a deadly virus (analysis showed 5000 different human-made toxic chemicals in the fat of dead seals!).

Some three-quarters of all cancer is caused by food, smoke and chemicals. Substances which have been shown to cause cancer in laboratory animals can be detoxified by enzymes in healthy human cells. By cleaning up our environment, in the home and outside, and by concentrating on building up our health, I think we could eliminate the majority of cancers without any more research, without any need to find a 'cure'.

Even animals get heart disease in stressful situations, and while every life is bound to have its share of difficulties and grief, the way we deal with painful situations has an important impact on our immune systems, and on whether or not we get ill. How do you cope with disappointment or loss? A desire to improve our health requires some thought about the social support network we have available – and about how willing we are to offer support to friends in need.

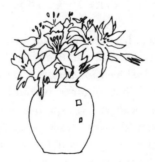

MAKING A HEALTHY HOME

The Green Home is a place where health is cultivated. A healthy environment is more than the sum of its parts – carefully filtered water and good ventilation doesn't make a house a home. Think hard about what makes your home alive, rich and stimulating and pleasurable. A really comfortable private place to sit down and read, or paint or frame pictures, is as important to creating a healthy home as switching to non-toxic cleaners.

Eating well is easier if you have the right foods on hand and get rid of unhealthy temptations. Move toxic cleaning and DIY products outside, into a garage or storeroom if possible, and get rid of cans of insecticides. Go through the bathroom cabinet, return old drugs to the chemist and separate non-prescription drugs you'd be better off without: laxatives, antacids (often high in aluminium), diuretics and aspirin. You won't necessarily feel happy about getting rid of these all at once, but you might put them in a box and see whether you can do without them for a month.

Start a safe medicine cabinet. I've found the following of value: aloe cream (or an aloe plant) for burns, calendula cream for cuts and skin irritations, and Olbas oil for colds. An adequate supply of bandages for emergencies is important, but taking a course in first aid is of more value than a vast range of gear.

SELF-CARE

A professional health assessment can be very useful, but even more important is your own assessment. Arrange an hour or so to yourself and consider the barriers to health in your life. Ask yourself questions: what condition is your hair in, your eyes, your skin? How is your hearing? Are you overweight or underweight? What about aches and pains, creaky joints? Don't restrict yourself to big worries which you would take to a doctor. What about athlete's foot or mouth ulcers, or even general stiffness? Don't assume that these things are the inevitable result of being human, or of growing old, and don't forget to look at good signs too.

Make a list as you go along. Do you feel tired all the time, or get depressed easily and for no particular reason? Trouble sleeping? Feelings of anger or aggression? Allergies or hay fever? Nervous mannerisms? Consider your job, the place you live, your relationships, your way of life. How satisfied are you? Can you laugh at yourself?

At the end of this you may have noted down two or three items – or you may have filled several pages. Of course you can't solve all these problems at once and you may need professional help for some of them. The key is to decide on one or two you really would like to sort out. Note them down and start thinking about what you can do about them.

If you are being treated by a doctor, find out as much as you can about the problem and about any medication you are taking. Make a list of questions and take it with you when you go to see the doctor. Change doctors if yours is reluctant to answer questions. If you are taking a course of prescription drugs and do not feel satisfied with the information you get from your doctor, go to a reference library and consult the *British National Formulary* (BNF), which lists all drugs used in the UK, with indications for use, contra-indications, effects and potential side effects. Consulting a practitioner of complementary medicine can be helpful when you need information about a chronic problem.

Instead of buying stronger glasses or contact lenses, try improving your eyesight. Ophthalmology places little or no emphasis on preventive treatment but eyes, like teeth, have regenerative capacity. Critics say that glasses act as a crutch, encouraging vision to deteriorate. Find out about Bates eye therapy teachers (see Sources).

STRESS MANAGEMENT

Virtually everyone who reads this is likely to be suffering from at least one stress-related symptom. Stress seems an inescapable part of modern life. A lot of minor stresses can add up to a large total stress burden and be just as hard on you as a serious catastrophe. Yet stress is not necessarily a bad thing. Much depends on how we respond to it – in fact, on our capacity for responding. The reason modern stresses seem to have an adverse effect may be that they are things outside our control or which we don't know how to change or respond to.

The suggestions for simplifying your life scattered through the book may help you think about ways to remove the causes of stress in your life. Here are a few more thoughts.

▶ Don't medicate stress. An estimated nine out of ten headaches are caused by tension, anxiety and other emotional states. Try a nap or a short walk, or a cup of hot sage or peppermint tea. Ask someone to rub your neck, or do some stretching exercises.

▶ Let go of relationships that create stress. Life is too short. Try to see more of the people who make you feel happy and energized.

▶ When you are stuck in traffic, late for a meeting or otherwise frustrated, take five deep breaths, smile at someone if possible and apply your mind to higher thoughts. Stress shortens your life expectancy. (If traffic is the problem, think about finding a job closer to home or plan to take the train next time.)

▶ Don't smoke and don't drink much.

▶ Stop taking dozens of vitamin supplements, and spend your money on delicious fresh fruit and vegetables instead.

▶ Get rid of fancy exercising equipment and walk.

▶ Get enough sleep, fresh air and natural light.

▶ Surround yourself with things and people you love.

NOISE

Whether you live in the centre of a large city or well outside the city limits, the volume of sound in your environment will have increased substantially over the past 70 years or so. For instance, the siren volume used by police and fire vehicles in urban areas has risen to 122 decibels, louder than a jet engine. Before the First World War a brass bell was enough to clear the road.

As a result, we do not hear as well as our ancestors. Loud sounds destroy sensory hair cells in the inner ear, and those do not regenerate. The process of hearing loss is gradual and cumulative, and we have come to expect it as a normal part of ageing. One study found that West Africans in their 70s had considerably better hearing than Londoners in the 20s.

Sound, for our ancestors, provided useful information about

the environment. Loud noises – the crack of thunder or falling rocks – were signs which helped them to deal with the world around. Most of the noise we face tells us nothing meaningful, but our bodies instinctively treat loud sounds as warning signals – our hearts beat faster, breathing speeds up and muscles tense. This reaction can lead to a wide range of health problems, from high blood pressure and headaches to ulcers, cardiovascular disease and disturbed sleep. Noise interferes with concentration and makes us raise our voices or turn the television up (increasing the overall noise level).

People who live near airports or busy motorways suffer from even louder 'normal' environments than inner city dwellers. European studies have shown that people living near an airport visit the doctor two or three times more often than average, suffer increased rates of high blood pressure, heart disease and psychological problems.

▶ Let noise be an important consideration when you choose a place to live (visit a prospective home at different times of day, during the week as well as at weekends).

▶ Plant hedges or rows of trees to muffle traffic noise.

▶ Use building features such as double pane glass, shutters, and solid doors, walls and floors to block out noise.

▶ Closets and cupboards built between rooms provide excellent soundproofing.

▶ Energy-saving insulation cuts down on noise as well as heat loss.

▶ Choose soft furnishings, lay carpets and put up cloth hangings.

▶ Choose quiet appliances and place rubber mats underneath noisy fridges, typewriters and other sources of domestic noise.

▶ Separate 'quiet' and 'noisy' rooms as much as possible.

▶ Place heavy furniture, like old-fashioned wooden wardrobes, against shared walls in flats or terraces.

▶ Turn down music (insist on the use of headphones if necessary).

▶ Wear protective ear covering when working with loud equipment, even an electric drill.

▶ Negotiate a music agreement – times of day and maximum levels on the volume control.

▶ Encourage pleasing sounds like music, falling water, wind in trees, chimes and birdsong.

EXERCISE

Think how ridiculous an aerobics class must seem to someone who gets all the exercise she needs hauling water from a well 3 miles away and growing the food for her family! We allocate special time for exercise because we lead sedentary lives. A simple switch from driving to walking or cycling can provide an adequate amount of exercise, probably enough to lower your chances of dropping dead of a heart attack at 55 substantially.

Instead of passive forms of recreation, why not think of hiking, cross-country skiing, swimming or cycling? 'Rambling' refreshes the mind as well as the body and provides city dwellers with much needed contact with the earth. (Driving through the countryside does not count as outdoor recreation!) Otherwise, find sports you enjoy, preferably outdoors so that you get light and fresh air along with the exercise. Sports centres are a discouraging development, with their artificial lighting, plastic food and the way they are geared to car owners, just like out-of-town shopping centres.

THE PECKHAM EXPERIMENT

Money does not buy good health. In fact the more doctors and drugs available to us, the more numerous the remedies, the more ill we seem to become. It seems that there is no time, no money and no inclination to keep people in a state of positive health, though the potential long-term financial savings would be considerable. Doctors get credit for ever more complex procedures rather than for their successes in cultivating a large number of healthy people.

In 1935 the Pioneer Health Centre was opened in Peckham, south-east London. Run as a family club, it was an experiment to discover, promote and study the growth of positive health. Each family was given an annual medical check-up, known as a 'health overhaul' and the findings were communicated at a family consultation. It combined the medical facilities, family planning, antenatal and postnatal clinics, nurseries for babies and pre-school children, leisure activities and a cafeteria. The building was especially designed for easy movement and visibility from one part to another. Families who lived in its catchment area were able to join this unique family club by paying a weekly fee. Members organized their own activities, and had a swimming pool and gym available. It was a place where leisure activities were as important as medical overhauls. Mothers shared in the preparation of the nursery teas and families spent many of their free hours at the centre.

Dr George Scott Williamson and Dr Innes Pearse were the co-founders and directors of the centre, and described it as an experiment into the nature of health. The emphasis was on cultivating health, as well as catching disease at an early stage by regular examinations.

The Peckham Centre closed during the war but was reopened in 1946 by public demand. The closure of the centre in 1950 was due to financial problems and the founding of the NHS. In social and research terms it was doing very well, with a membership of almost 900 families.

Perhaps now is the time to look at its principles again. Instead of focusing attention and praise on curing rare diseases, and on treating ever-increasing numbers of patients, we would all benefit from a decentralized service which catered for a wider interpretation of human health.

COMPLEMENTARY MEDICINE

Orthodox medicine is beginning to accept, albeit reluctantly, that alternative treatments are popular and often effective. The Health Education Authority (HEA) issues a *Guide to Complementary Medicine and Therapies*, rating different approaches for medical credibility, scientific research, availability and popularity. In a recent survey, three-quarters of respondents wanted to have alternative therapies available on the NHS. Three out of ten British people – in a population of 58 million – have used alternative therapies, and some GPs now refer patients to the more accepted alternative practitioners – acupuncturists, osteopaths and hypnotherapists. With public demand for their services growing by an estimated 20 per cent each year, complementary – or alternative or non-conventional – practitioners are becoming a significant part of our health care system.

Holistic medicine aims to treat the whole person, not just a symptom. Many holistic practitioners do not like to think in terms of 'disease'. Instead, they describe a particular set of symptoms as a common pattern of coping responses. The actual cause, which is what they want to deal with, may be different for each person. The way each person responds to his or her physical and social environment is different. Every treatment needs to be individually tailored. This sort of analysis takes more time than a typical surgery visit to your doctor (or the five minutes you are booked with a hospital consultant), and a first visit to an alternative practitioner is likely to take an hour or so because you will be asked to discuss your health history and way of life.

■How To Choose A Practitioner

Seeing an acupuncturist or an osteopath generally means spending your hard-earned cash and you'll want to make a careful selection, both of a particular person and of a speciality. Most people rely on friends for advice, but you can also consult the HEA guide and specific licensing bodies. If you don't have much money, talk to the practitioner about reduced fees or even offer to barter some skill of your own for treatment.

Going to a group practice is a good idea because you can easily be passed on to someone else if the person you first consult feels that this is appropriate. A good alternative therapist will be aware of other disciplines and happy to make referrals. Beware anyone who think their own speciality is the only way. Look for a practitioner who makes you feel comfortable, who is enthusiastic and encouraging, and who clearly takes an individual approach to your health problem. A willingness to explain the treatment and to enlist your support is important, as is confidence in the body's ability to heal itself.

In many alternative fields, there is no legal restriction on who is qualified to practise. There are, however, bodies which accredit schools and award particular qualifications, and you would be well advised to consult one of these before choosing a practitioner (see Sources).

DYING GREEN

We have come to accept a medically monitored death in hospital, followed by cremation and floral tributes, as the usual, and even desirable, thing. Dying is part of living and the way people end their lives should be part of all our lives, marked by dignity, and within a community of friends and family. Tragically, an increasing number of people end their lives alone in a hospital bed, with none of their own things, no familiar faces, to look at and cherish.

Why has death become institutionalized? Because we want to give the dying every possible chance, because we want modern medicine to make death go away, or because we do not want to have to come to terms with death, with our own future deaths? The hospice movement is an excellent sign of better understanding about the needs of the dying, when being at home isn't possible. Pain relief and nursing care are often all that someone needs as they end their days, along with a homelike atmosphere, the care and attention of friends or family, and perhaps spiritual succour. A proper environment for dying, and a restoration of the dignity of those who are near to death, is an important part of understanding and accepting ecological life cycles.

And after death, there are choices to be made. More and more people who care about the natural world are reluctant to think of polluting it after their death, with chemical treatment of the body, polluting smoke from a crematorium, and non-biodegradable coffins and funeral trappings. The Natural Death Centre publishes a guide to green burial, and a number of councils around Britain have set aside land near existing graveyards for 'woodland cemeteries'. The Institute of Burial and Cremation Administration finds that these options are attractive to many people, and the trend seems likely to grow. There are surprisingly few legal restrictions on burial: you do not have to have a coffin, a gravestone, an undertaker or a religious ceremony.

In Carlisle, future residents can choose to be buried in a biodegradable cardboard coffin or in a locally woven woollen burial shroud. Graves are generally unmarked, though sometimes a small plaque can be posted. An oak sapling and several hundred bluebell bulbs are planted on each grave and wildflower seeds are scattered. Think of it: you can help to reforest Britain and make this land a green and pleasant one, long after your days of fighting motorway construction are done.

12

THE NON-TOXIC HOME

Since the Second World War there has been a staggering increase in the number of human-made chemical substances in common use. The majority of them have not been adequately tested for risk to human health or the environment. Products we use every day contain chemicals which are known to be carcinogenic (cancer causing), mutagenic (mutation causing) and teratogenic ('monster' causing – that is, leading to birth defects). Toxic chemicals from industry, accidentally released into the environment or 'disposed' of, pose an increasing threat.

Chemicals cause cancer, miscarriages and birth defects, and in the longer term affect the human gene pool. They also have subtle, low-level effects, and a growing number of people find themselves sensitive to food additives and colourings, chlorine bleach, enzyme detergents and other chemical products. Things which are hazardous to human health are almost always hazardous to the outside environment. The detergents, bleach and disinfectant we pour down the drain find their way into our lakes and rivers, where their 'powerful cleansing action' has a devastating effect on water plants and animal life, and some eventually ends up back in our food or in the water we drink.

Toxic waste is a growing problem in the industrialized world. By-products of chemical production are, at present levels, impossible to deal with safely. The Health and Safety Executive recently condemned the inadequate safety procedures at some of Britain's most hazardous industrial sites, and according to the UN Environment Programme (UNEP), 'International chemical trade involved almost all sectors of society'. The UNEP has developed a code of ethics for chemical production and management, which, they say, must take account of the entire life cycle with the explicit purpose of reducing the health and environmental risks posed by human-made chemicals.

Domestic rubbish also has its share of toxic contaminants. Think how casually we throw away used batteries, an old box of moth balls or a couple of cans of dried-up paint. A few councils have special toxic waste collection points, but most of us have no choice about how to discard these items. The main thing we can do, individually, is to try to stop using toxic products, and to encourage the producers of environmentally benign alternatives.

ECOLOGICAL CONNECTIONS

While a few people react to the dyes and fragrances in commercial toilet paper, we need to be aware that all bleached paper – white loo rolls, kitchen towels, facial tissues, coffee filters and so on – has been found to contain traces of the highly toxic chemical dioxin. This is the result of standard pulping and bleaching operations, and because the chemicals are also released in large quantities into lakes and rivers, paper mills are one of the most polluting of industries. For alternatives, see Chapter 4, pp. 59–61.

Women will be especially interested to know about recent research into the environmental causes of breast cancer. High oestrogen levels have been linked to known risk factors such as early menstruation, late menopause, not bearing a child or bearing one late in life, but it was assumed that because this was a matter of hormones women had little control over it. Organochlorines are chlorine-based chemical compounds in wide use throughout the world. They include DDT (still in use in some places, and still turning up traces in our food), PCBs and dioxins, as well as commonly used herbicides, fungicides, germicides, preservatives and solvents. They mimic the effects of oestrogen and accumulate particularly in fatty tissue. These chemical effects are sometimes passed down from generation to generation. There are an increasing number of health disorders being seen in the children and grandchildren of people exposed to particular hazards.

It is virtually impossible to test the effects of individual chemicals on human beings. The so-called 'chemical cocktail' – the wide variety of chemicals we are exposed to in our food, air, water, building materials and domestic products – may well have serious consequences. There is no way to test the effects of each possible combination of chemicals. Judging safe levels is equally difficult, and recommendations are frequently lowered as scientists discover more about the way particular chemicals affect human beings.

This chapter offers a brief overview of an increasingly complex subject and concentrates on the practicalities of choosing non-toxic alternatives.

CHEMICAL SENSITIVITY

While our bodies are able to deal with a certain quantity of environmental poisons, each person's chemical tolerance point is different. Once it has been passed, severe and debilitating illness can result.

Sometimes removing a proportion of the environmental toxins can enable coping mechanisms to function again, but it seems that certain people become permanently sensitive even to things which they were previously able to tolerate. Possible symptoms include asthma and eczema, depression, chronic fatigue, skin rashes and migraine headaches.

Sensitive individuals find that pesticide residues on fresh fruits and vegetables, traces of detergent and solvents in and on many products, and a wide variety of additives make them ill. Reactions to petrochemical products are common.

Children take in more air and more food for their body weight than do adults, and are more vulnerable to environmental toxins, just as they are to ionizing radiation. Allergies, including asthma and eczema, seem to be more and more common, and children's reactions to chemicals can include hyperactivity and even psychiatric disorders.

Pregnant women, and their unborn babies, are also particularly vulnerable to chemical toxins. Whatever they consume or come into contact with will affect, to some degree, their baby. If you are pregnant, make a special effort to avoid contact with strong household chemicals, particularly aerosols. Watch out with cosmetics as well. Chemical hair colourings and hair sprays, and of course smoking, are thought to be the greatest danger to the foetus.

Low-level chemical exposure influences each one of us. Do you feel light-headed when you use spray adhesives or queasy in a newly-painted room? Many people are sensitive to washing powders and 'original formula, no enzyme' detergents are promoted almost as vigorously as their 'biological' cousins.

THE CLEAN HOME

Take a look at the variety of cleaners you have in your house. How many do you actually use? Spray polishes and carpet fresheners are enticingly packaged and expensively promoted, and advertisements about laundry powders are inescapable.

One reason we are so prone to try new products is that few of us devote substantial amounts of time to house cleaning, and we're eager to try anything that might make the job easier and faster. We buy the promise rather than the product and end up with a cupboard full of fat, luridly-coloured plastic bottles – each used once or twice and then superseded by the next bright aerosol to catch our eye.

Rather than buy more, why not keep a supply of basic cleaning products which will harm neither you nor the environment? Virtually all cleaning chores can be efficiently tackled with nothing more than soap, vinegar and bicarbonate of soda (this may sound extreme, but please read on). You can also buy safe commercial cleaners.

Switching to non-toxic toiletries is even simpler because there are more commercial products available. It is also possible to make your own non-toxic alternatives.

Don't think that anything which calls itself 'natural' will be. 'Natural' wild-mountain-honey-and-herb shampoo may contain exactly the same ingredients as any other detergent shampoo, with the addition of a little honey and a different fragrance. Full product labelling is an important step towards offering consumers an informed choice.

Household products are designed to clean, to disinfect and to deodorize. To achieve these aims we use vast quantities of detergent, bleach, air fresheners and other dangerous products.

None of us wants to go back to great-granny's days of scrubbing clothes on a washboard or scouring floors with ashes. But non-toxic cleaning is easy, and there are fewer supplies to think about. Non-toxic products seem to take far less rinsing (and you don't have to worry about traces of bleach or ammonia left behind).

We use too many cleaning products and far too much of them. The first and best cleaner is water, and a good rule of thumb is 'eliminate – saturate – absorb'. Rather than grinding away at the pudding batter that has dried on to your cooker, simply wet everything with a soapy dishcloth and leave it alone for ten minutes. Then wipe it up. If there are a few spots left, you can always scrub them. This principle works on clothes (soak overnight) and floors (wet the floor and leave for half an hour – you'll be amazed at the amount of dirt which comes up), as well as on dishes.

Another useful hint, for all of us who want to avoid both chemical cleaning products and cleaning in the first place, is to use good doormats at every door. Carpets last longer if they are kept clean – it's the abrasiveness of dirt, rather than traffic, which does most of the damage. In addition, mats will cut down on the pollutants, including lead and canine parasites, you bring into the house. (But don't shake them on to the garden or you'll end up eating the lead in next year's lettuces.) Taking your shoes off when you come in works the same magic.

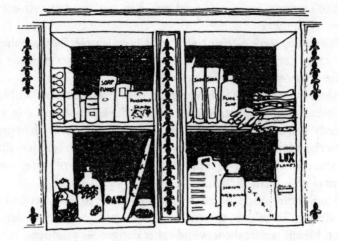

THE ECOLOGICAL CLEANING CUPBOARD

Here is a list of basic supplies which should get you through every domestic task. They are unscented but you can add a few drops of essential oil to create your own fresh and naturally clean smell. Look out for containers which can be reused to package your basic cleaning supplies. Shakers are useful for bicarbonate of soda and borax, and spray bottles are good for a window cleaning mixture.

■Soap

Household soap or plain soap flakes will do the trick much of the time, perhaps with the addition of a little washing soda. And a constant refrain in books on housekeeping and saving money is the soap jar – this is where all those slivers of hand soap belong, while you start a fresh bar. Pour on a little boiling water and you'll get a soft jelly which can be used for washing dishes or tights or diluted as a spray for aphids. Another way to use soap scraps is to keep them in a metal tea ball or strainer, which you swish in your washing-up water.

■Washing-up Liquid

You may not need this, if you become a soap jar *aficionado*. But Ecover's biodegradable version smells delicious, is effective and truly easy on hands. Faith Products Clear Spring washing-up liquid is another good one (it contains lemon grass and citrus extracts to cut grease, and is completely vegan). In a hard water area, add a little water softener to the wash basin – you'll need less soap.

■Laundry Powder

A number of biodegradable washing powders are available from wholefood stores, some supermarkets and by mail order. You may need to add a water softener to get clothes clean in hard water.

People used to air clothes overnight and get another day's wear out of them – you'll know yourself whether this will work! Brushing (with a good natural bristle clothes brush) is the butler's trick for reviving woollen garments. Machine washing and tumble drying make clothes wear out more quickly. See below, p. 200 for more on clothes care.

■Bicarbonate Of Soda

Almost infinitely useful around the house. Buy a 500 g box from the chemist rather than the tiny ones you get for baking. It is a partial water softener, can be used as a scouring powder on sinks and baths (effective and very easy to rinse away), as a coating on ovens (to make them easier to clean next time), an excellent polish for chrome and a neutral cleaner when dissolved in water. Bicarbonate of soda also makes a good plaque-fighting toothpowder, and can be used in solution as a garden fungicide for mildew on roses and other plants (2 g per litre of water, applied every seven days).

■Table Salt

Salt is mildly disinfectant and makes an abrasive but benign scouring powder. Keep drains clear with a weekly handful of salt and kettleful of boiling water.

■Tea Tree Oil

This natural disinfectant from Australia is an ideal addition to the ecological cleaning cupboard. It kills germs and has a strong, clean smell which will satisfy people who want the bathroom to 'smell' clean.

■Borax

Borax is a natural mineral product that kills germs and mildew. An American hospital tested a borax solution as a disinfectant and found that it satisfied their germicidal requirements. Use it to soak nappies, whiten clothes, soften water and increase the effectiveness of plain soap. It is also good at keeping down mould and preventing odours.

■White Distilled Vinegar

Mix with water (see below, pp. 195–6) to make a cleaner for glass and tiles. Use to descale your kettle or remove stains from a teapot. Mixed with salt or baking soda, it will polish brass and copper.

■Water Softener

A softener will improve washing results and enable you to cut down on the amount of powder you use. (When you switch to a biodegradable powder, run your clothes through a wash cycle with a double dose of water softener to remove detergent residue.) It can also be used as a bath salt, with the addition of a scented oil or fresh herbs.

Scented products are often implicated in allergic reactions, so buy a softener with no added fragrance. Boots makes one which is a blend of sodium bicarbonate and sodium carbonate, or use ordinary washing soda.

■Washing Soda

This is a water softener and cuts grease. Used sparingly, this makes a good heavy duty cleaner for walls and floors, and a few tablespoons added to your regular washing powder will help with really dirty clothes.

■Trisodium Phosphate (TSP)

TSP is a powerful and moderately toxic cleaner sometimes available from paint shops (this is the active ingredient in the powder you buy to clean walls before painting). Try to buy it 'straight' rather than mixed with detergents and fragrance. It is a phosphate and therefore has a harmful effect on water supplies, but chemically sensitive people find it useful as it gives off no fumes. Use only when absolutely necessary and wear rubber gloves.

■Furniture Polish

The National Trust Book of Housekeeping (Penguin, 1993) says that you should *never* use aerosol polishes, especially those containing silicone. Aerosols give instant shine but do not fill in scratches and make the furniture surface slippery. Continued use leads to a milky finish, because of the solvents they contain, which can only be removed by stripping and refinishing the piece of furniture. The authors advise using a hard furniture polish once, or at most twice, a year. In between, just dust or rub with a soft cloth, not a feather duster. A slightly dampened cloth will remove sticky marks and a little vinegar in the water will cut old polish film.

Make your own beeswax polish by grating beeswax (from the chemist or your own beehive) into a jar and covering it with natural turpentine. Shake occasionally until the beeswax has dissolved.

A revitalizing liquid polish can be made by combining two parts boiled linseed oil and one part turpentine. Buy both at a DIY shop (don't try boiling your own linseed oil). Applied sparingly and rubbed in well, this is suggested as an alternative to refinishing a piece of furniture.

■Floor Polish

A hard, traditional carnauba wax is appropriate for fine wood floors. Many people get by perfectly well without waxing or polishing their floors at all. Linoleum will survive nicely with an occasional mopping with soapy water.

■Cleaning Cloths And Scourers

Those round knitted nylon scourers last for ever. Choose cellulose rather than plastic sponges (you can cut up the large ones sold for cars into manageable pieces), and accumulate cotton cleaning and polishing rags. Linen is best for glass. A metal scourer can stand in for a lot of scouring powder. Use plain steel wool rather than steel wool pads – you can tear off the small piece which is all you really need and choose your own soap.

Mail order sources of non-allergenic and biodegradable cleaning products, toiletries, vitamins and minerals are listed at the back of the book, and it is worth looking for commercial products aimed at the chemically sensitive. Boots, for example, has a range of cleaning supplies which contain no perfumes or colourants, and the ingredients have been selected for their low irritancy. These are likely to be less polluting than other commercial products.

AN A–Z OF CLEANING TIPS

Brass: according to *The National Trust Book of Housekeeping*, brass fittings on furniture should not be shiny – just well rubbed along with the wood. Lemon juice or white vinegar mixed with bicarbonate of soda will polish brass articles, as will ketchup and even Worcestershire sauce!

Burnt pans: fill with water and add a good handful of salt. Soak overnight, after bringing to a boil if the burning is very bad.

Carpets: combine one part washing-up liquid with four parts boiling water. Allow to cool and whip to a foam with an egg beater. Sponge into carpet and wipe away with a damp cloth. You can use a steam-cleaning machine with plain water. For gentle cleaning and deodorizing, sprinkle carpet heavily with a mixture of one part borax to two parts maize meal, or with plain bicarbonate of soda (use lots). Leave for an hour or two, then vacuum. Snow also makes a good cleaner, if you have some available, because it doesn't wet the carpet too much.

Heavy-duty cleaners: use washing soda or TSP, but cautiously. A completely natural and non-toxic product is available through catering suppliers: a simple pumice bar which is recommended for all durable surfaces, including tiles.

Ovens: first, try to keep the oven reasonably clean. Use steel wool after thoroughly wetting the oven walls and allowing the dirt to soften. Wipe the newly cleaned oven with a solution of one heaped tablespoon of bicarbonate of soda to half a pint of water, to make the task far easier next time.

Scouring powder: instead of the commercial products, which contain bleach, use plain bicarbonate of soda on a sponge. It works beautifully and is good for shining chrome fittings. (It can, however, scratch plexiglass or perspex; if in doubt, test on a corner first.) Fine wood ash can be used and horsetail is an excellent natural scourer. This plant grows in the wild (railway embankments are a good place to look) and its fine silica do the work.

Silver: can be soaked for 10–15 minutes or gently simmered in a saucepan containing hot water, a few aluminium milk bottle tops or a piece of foil and one tablespoon of washing soda. A little toothpaste will polish jewellery, but for really delicate pieces try pure alcohol (or surgical spirit) on a fine paint brush.

Tiles: if you apply a wax polish to clean tiles, they will be easy to wipe down. Scrubbing with bicarbonate of soda on a sponge is effective on water spots as is a 50/50 vinegar and water mixture.

Toilets: bleach only oxidizes toilet stains, rather than removing them, and it is hard on chrome and formica. The ring in your toilet comes from hard water (just the same as the limescale in the kettle) and can be removed with an acid like vinegar, left to stand. I find that the easiest solution is occasionally scrubbing with a piece of wet-and-dry sandpaper, although this does scratch the ceramic glaze. Use a mild borax or tea tree oil solution to disinfect.

Windows: mix two tablespoons of white vinegar with two cups of water and a few drops of liquid soap in a spray bottle. Polish with clean, lint-free cotton or linen rags, or ordinary newspaper. Cold tea and newspaper also works well. If you've been using commercial glass cleaners you may find a waxy build-up from your old spray. Wipe down with a little surgical spirit or washing soda to remove the film.

WHAT ABOUT GERMS?

There is too much scaremongering about household germs. Germs are just bacteria and bacteria are all around us. What we should aim for is a clean, sweet-smelling place to live, where potentially hazardous bacteria (generally from food or other human beings) is controlled by basic hygiene. In general, hospitals are the only places where people get sick from bacteria on doorknobs, because hospitals have truly dangerous bacteria in them. A healthy human immune system can easily cope with normal household germs and is in fact at greater risk from the chemicals in many cleaning products.

Natural disinfectants include borax, tea tree oil, grapefruit seed oil and other citrus extracts.

AIR FRESHENING

Don't equate the smell of bleach or other harsh cleaners with freshness. For chemically-sensitive people and people with allergies, including asthma, the smell of ammonia or disinfectant can be debilitating. Quite a few people seem to regard commercial air fresheners as part of good hygiene around the house (80 per cent of UK households use them), but they work by masking unpleasant odours, coating your nasal passages with an oily film or numbing your sense of smell with a nerve-deadening agent. Most air fresheners do nothing to freshen the air, they merely add more pollutants. Try these ideas instead.

1. Plenty of ventilation. Open windows, at least once a day, are the best way to clear stale or offensive odours, as well as any toxic fumes which might build up. An extractor fan can help in the kitchen and bathroom.

2. Keep things dry and reasonably warm. Clothes should be aired thoroughly. Borax inhibits the growth of mildew and mould, so you can sprinkle it around or wipe surfaces with a borax solution.

3. Empty your rubbish frequently and sprinkle a little borax or bicarbonate of soda in the bottom of the bin. (Once you start composting, your rubbish bin stays dry and is very unlikely to smell.)

4. Compost buckets should be emptied every couple of days and probably every day in the summer. A cover keeps flies away.

There are a number of ideas for natural, and delightful, air fresheners in Chapter 9.

HOUSEHOLD PESTS

Insecticides are poisonous, and should be avoided both because of their environmental effects and effects of our health. First, remove whatever is attracting the pests. Food should be stored in air-tight containers (glass jars are excellent) and take special care with cleaning. Wash up dishes immediately after eating, don't leave crumbs, and empty wastebaskets frequently. Try the following suggestions.

∎ Ants

Sprinkle dried mint, chilli powder or borax wherever they are coming in – of course, your first step should be to block the hole, if possible. Plant mint outside; ants don't like the smell.

∎ Cockroaches

Try baking them out – heating the house as hot as it will get for a couple of hours. Easier, and safer, is to leave out a mixture of flour, cocoa and borax, or bicarbonate of soda and powdered sugar, or flour and plaster of Paris (out of the reach of children, of course). All of these should lead to a quick death for the noxious creatures. Another method is to make a 'trap' by putting a few sweets in the bottom of a glass jar, with a bit of wood for a ramp. They climb in but cannot get out.

∎ Flies

Hang bunches of bay leaves, mint, pennyroyal or eucalyptus by your doors. Old-fashioned sticky fly paper is safe and effective, if gruesome. Make your own by soaking strips of heavy brown paper in a thick sugar syrup. Let them dry until just sticky to the touch, then hang in out of the way places. You can put the following mixture into little cloth bags and hang them over doors: equal parts of dried and crushed bay leaves, pennyroyal, ground cloves and eucalyptus leaves, very slightly dampened with eucalyptus oil. Citrus oil is another repellant and fly swatters are effective.

∎ Lice

The plague of schoolchildren and their families. Environmentalists suspect that the resurgence of this problem may be the result of over use of pesticides, which have encouraged the creepy-crawlies to mutate into ever more resistant forms. The most effective and safe method of removal is thorough combing. While we don't like having such intimate contact with such distasteful creatures, excessively strong pesticide solutions and shampoo are not a good long-term solution. Schools are alert to the problem and you should be, too. The earlier lice are spotted the easier they are to deal with. Read shampoo labels and choose those which are pyrethrum-based. This is a natural insecticide derived from chrysanthemums, less toxic than other products. Environmental specialists recommend coconut oil and coconut oil based shampoos to kill lice, too, but careful combing is still necessary to remove the eggs.

■Moths

Mothballs are made of paradichlorobenzene, a volatile chemical which is a respiratory irritant, and can cause depression, seizures and long-term damage to kidneys and liver. Although the packet may warn 'avoid prolonged breathing of vapour', the way mothballs are used (distributed among your clothing) makes prolonged exposure unavoidable. Cedar wood, lavender and natural camphor are natural, traditional moth repellants but the most important thing is to ensure that woollens are cleaned before being stored. Pressing with a steam iron or tumbling in a dryer will also kill any moth eggs. I know people who swear by scented soap, packed with woollens.

■Insect Repellants

Rather than apply commercial repellants, which contain Deet (diethyl toluamide), a strong irritant which can eat through plastic and dissolve paint, rub your skin with vinegar (on a cotton wool ball) and allow to dry. The smell disappears as it dries, but makes you taste nasty. Or rub on oil of citronella or pennyroyal diluted in a little vegetable oil. Citronella candles are standard insect repellants in the US.

CLOTHES CARE

Modern washing powders are detergents, with a variety of additives including optical brighteners, enzymes and fragrances. All of these have environmental and health effects, as well as disputed effects on your clothes. Major companies aim to out-do one another with new ingredients and whiter washes.

Some of the problems associated with detergent use are explained in Chapter 10. Instead, there are biodegradable, enzyme-free products available from various suppliers. Before you switch to a washing powder which does not contain optical brighteners, it may help to run your clothes through a wash cycle with a double dose of softener. Otherwise they can turn slightly yellow because of detergent film. On the other hand, they may simply be returning to their natural colour. To make your own washing powder, combine 1 cup soap flakes and $^1/_2$ cup washing soda. In soft water areas you can use a higher proportion of soap flakes and in hard water areas you'll need more washing soda.

If you're hooked on spot spray, try rubbing clothes with a damp bar of household soap or use this home-made spot spray: $^1/_2$ cup ammonia, $^1/_2$ cup white vinegar, $^1/_4$ cup baking soda, 2 tablespoons liquid soap and 1 pint water. Simpler yet, presoak in plain water or in soapy wash water. Use the prewash cycle or just switch the machine off after it has filled and leave it for a couple of hours or overnight, then wash as usual.

■Whiteners

Find alternatives to bleach, because it is a dangerous product which should not be used routinely. I've been trying to find an oxygen (rather than chlorine) bleach for clothes, but with no success. These have been on the market in the US for a number of years and we may see them in the UK before long. Water softeners are useful alternatives. With very delicate fabrics, presoak for 10–30 minutes in a mixture of 1 part hydrogen peroxide to 7 parts water.

Hanging out on a line in the sunshine is good for whitening

clothes. An old method was to spread them on green vegetation – a lawn, for example – as the oxygen produced by the plants is said to be helpful. Boiling sounds prehistoric to anyone who wasn't brought up in an era when teatowels were boiled daily. But as long as you have a large soup pot, it is easy enough and certainly effective. I'm not suggesting that we go back to routinely boiling clothes, but as an occasional treat for white cottons, why not? Allow to cool, drain off most of the water and spin in your washing machine or spin dryer. (Remember that this will only work with 100 per cent cotton or linen – not polyester blends!)

■Fabric Conditioners

Conditioners, or softeners, were designed for use with synthetic fabrics, to prevent static cling. If you are using natural fibre fabrics, this shouldn't be a problem. In a hard water area they do seem to give softer handwashed woollens, but a little white vinegar (soak a few dried herbs in it if you want a pleasant fragrance) should do the trick – and running a warm iron over the dry jumper also softens it.

Or mix one part bicarbonate of soda, one part white or herbal vinegar and two parts water. Use as you would a commercial fabric softener. Ecover's fabric softener is made of natural fatty acids, water and lemon oil, and is biodegradable.

People often use softeners to make clothes smell 'fresh'. Hanging them outside does a far better job and you don't have to worry about possible allergic reactions. Artificial fragrances do not freshen anything. If you cannot dry outside, how about herbal bags in your drawers and cupboards?

■Ironing

Rather than use spray starch in an aerosol can, with their inherent dangers, try one or more of the following ideas.

1. You can still buy old-fashioned starch, which you mix up with cold water, and then add boiling water and stir to a smooth paste. This is obviously more complicated than using

an aerosol spray. But just how many of your clothes really need to be starched? It's fun to give linen napkins and lace collars an occasional stiff starching, but 100 per cent cotton and linen have a naturally crisp finish after ironing. It is synthetic fabrics which tend to need perking up with starch.

2. Mix starch powder (or even ordinary cornflour) with water in a sprayer. Add a little cologne or a few drops of an essential oil if you want it scented. A rounded tablespoon of starch to 1 pint of water will give an average hold. (I prefer to mix the starch with boiling water, according to package directions, and then dilute.) Shake before spraying and wipe the nozzle with a damp cloth when you finish – but don't keep for long or it will grow amazingly mouldy!

3. Try taking your freshly laundered garments to a dry cleaning establishment for pressing-only with their special high-temperature equipment. Many cleaners will do this – ring around.

■Dry Cleaning

'Dry' cleaning is done by using a solvent instead of water to wash clothes. The industry has a history of fatal worker illness as a result of the chemicals used. Carbon tetrachloride was used until recently, but was found to cause cancer. The most common solvents used currently are two organochlorines, trichlorotrifluoroethane and perchloroethylene. They, too, are toxic, and the former is a chlorofluorohydrocarbon, one of the CFCs causing the deterioration of the ozone layer. Short-term, acute exposure can cause giddiness, nausea and unconsciousness. Chronic exposure is even worse because the compounds accumulate in body tissue, and lead to organ damage and cancer risk. Prolonged exposure to perchloroethylene can cause breast and liver cancer.

Although dry cleaning chemicals evaporate after a short time, the environmental consequences of manufacturing, transporting and disposing of them mean that we should avoid dry cleaning as much as possible. We should also consider whether we want to pay for other people to spend their days working with such hazardous chemicals.

The best possible advice is not to buy clothes that are difficult or even hazardous to clean. I have washed dozens of garments labelled 'Dry clean only' by hand or machine. (Manufacturers do not want to be held responsible for careless washing by the customer and sometimes use these labels as precautionary measures.) Wash cotton garments in the machine, and silk and wool by hand. Use a mild soap – Lux Flakes or Ecover Wool Wash, for example, or soft soap made with soap scraps – and add a little vinegar to the rinse water to cut soap film. Sweater should be squeezed out in a towel, then dried flat, and silks should be allowed to drip dry, then ironed while still slightly damp.

The clothes that do require special treatment are tailored clothes with many layers of different fabrics in lining and interlining. If you do have clothes dry cleaned, ensure that they are thoroughly aired, outdoors or in an unoccupied room, before being put away.

The US Environmental Protection Agency has been studying 'wet cleaning' in an effort to reduce exposure to hazardous dry cleaning chemicals. This new washing process does not require solvents. They are finding that the initial investment to get a shop going is lower than that for dry cleaning and customers prefer wet-cleaned clothes because they smell better.

■ Stain Removal

Dry cleaning fluid, like dry cleaning, should be avoided. Complicated advice on dealing with stains is lost on most modern housekeepers, but a simple range of products should enable you to deal with most domestic crises.

The most important thing to remember is to start with cold water, particularly on protein-based spots like blood, egg or gravy. Hot water will cook and set the stain, and you'll probably never get it out.

1.   The standard trick of pouring salt on a wine stain is usually

effective, and is also worth trying on fruit and beetroot stains.

2. Getting out the soda syphon (or just a bottle of whatever fizzy water you drink, or plain soda water) works on many stains.

3. A borax solution – one part borax to eight parts water – is worth keeping handy (out of the reach of children) for treating a wide range of stains. Sponge it on and let it dry, before washing with soap and cold water.

4. Plain old boiling water is good for fruit and tea stains – preferably poured on taut fabric from a great height (centre the spot over a bowl and stretch it tight with an elastic band, put it in the bath and start pouring).

5. Rub grass stains with glycerine (from the chemist) before washing. It is brilliant on cricket trousers and worth trying on cosmetic stains. You may need to follow with washing soda to remove the oily element of the stain.

6. Eucalyptus oil (from the chemist) will deal with nasties like tar and oil and grass stains. Rub it in well, then wash as normal. An effective tar remover is lard (or another solid fat), thoroughly rubbed in and then washed out – use some washing soda to cut the grease.

7. Soak perspiration stains in water with a good dollop of white vinegar or a handful of bicarbonate of soda – try both and see which works for you. This apparently depends on your particular body chemistry.

8. Try lemon juice and salt on rust stains, then lay in the sunshine for a couple of days. Clothes used to be 'bleached' in this way as they dried over bushes or on the clothesline. It both whitens and deodorizes, and the clothes smell wonderful. It is worth trying on even the most impossible of stains, and is essential for cloth nappies.

NON-TOXIC GARDENING

- Treat all hazardous DIY and cleaning products as if they could cause cancer: use them sparingly, ventilate well, keep them away from children and invalids, and don't flush them down the lavatory.
- Buy only what you absolutely need and cannot find a substitute for.
- Read warning labels and follow directions, erring on the side of caution.
- Don't use more than the directions call for, and you might even start with a bit less.
- Close containers tightly.
- Work outside if possible and try not to breathe in fumes – take ventilation seriously. (Wear a thick sweater and keep the windows open.)
- Do not mix chemicals (bleach and ammonia are a potentially deadly combination, and many cleaning products contain one or the other).
- Wear protective clothing and a mask if necessary, and protect your hands with rubber gloves.
- Avoid wearing soft contact lenses while working with any solvent.
- Clean up carefully, both yourself and your work area.
- Store in the original container (don't leave white spirit in an unlabelled jam jar, for example).
- Try to use up what you've bought. Dispose of any leftovers through a hazardous waste programme, should your council have one, or carefully sealed and wrapped in the dustbin – not down the drain!
- Keep dangerous chemicals well out of children's reach.

THE NON-TOXIC OFFICE

An increasing number of us spend most of our waking hours in an office, and a rapidly growing percentage of people have offices at home. Here are a number of ways to reduce your impact on the environment and make your office a healthier place to spend your days.

▶ Declare your office a no smoking area.
▶ Use water-based correction fluid and odourless water-based marker pens.
▶ Use latex rather than oil based paint.
▶ Switch from halon fire extinguishers to carbon dioxide ones.
▶ Use green cleaning products and rechargeable batteries.
▶ Have your printing done with soya ink on recycled paper.
▶ Place photocopying machines at a distance from desks and work stations.

DIY PRODUCTS

Finding substitutes for potentially hazardous building and decorating materials is a difficult issue. Information and safe products are discussed in Chapter 6. But we all need to use hazardous products on occasion. Take a close look at warning labels, choose the least toxic products, and use them sparingly and carefully. See pages 96–7 for clean up tips.

AVOIDING PLASTICS

In Chapter 3, we looked at the ecological problem posed by our excessive use of plastics. Plastics also pose a problem for human health. Many plastics out-gas throughout their use. You won't be conscious of this except with something like a brand new shower curtain (if you can smell it, it is out-gassing), but plastics do add to the total level of air pollutants. Synthetic fabrics continually give off fine fibres which go into the air, and some researchers believe that the rise in juvenile asthma and allergies is associated with the increased use of man-made materials in homes and schools.

PVC (polyvinyl chloride) plastic, for example, is extremely common, used for everything from tablecloths to shoe soles, and credit cards to squeezy toys. It is made with vinyl chloride, a chemical recognized as causing cancer, birth defects, skin diseases and liver dysfunction, as well as other health problems. PVC is somewhat unstable, especially if it contains added plasticizers.

Plastics are not going to go away, and they are undeniably useful for certain purposes. It is possible, however, to reduce the plastics in your home by choosing to buy products made from natural materials. Look for wooden toys, rattan waste baskets, leather or cotton canvas shoes, pottery mixing bowls, and natural cotton and wool bedding.

NON-TOXIC LIVING SIMPLIFIED

- Choose patterned carpets and furnishings so that occasional spots and duelling wounds won't be noticed.
- Choose dark-coloured and patterned fabrics whenever possible.
- Make or buy unlined curtains and washable slipcovers for furniture.
- Assume that hazardous DIY and cleaning products cause cancer and use them accordingly!
- If you don't want people to use certain noxious products around you or your children, the most tactful reason to give is that you're allergic.

13

REDUCING RADIATION

For months after the Chernobyl disaster in 1986 we were all suddenly conscious of our vulnerability to radiation and its peculiarly frightening nature. We wondered if it was safe to go outdoors or to drink the milk from our doorsteps. We asked one another if we could trust the government experts who sallied forth on every news bulletin to reassure us that all was well. There are many nuclear power stations closer to home, but Chernobyl made it abundantly clear that distance provides no safeguard and that the threat of radiation is a terrifying development of the modern age.

Even as we approach a decade after the disaster at Chernobyl, farmers in Norway must take special steps to lower radiation in their livestock – an ironic and bitter state of affairs because Norway has long banned nuclear plants but is forced to spend millions every year monitoring and dealing with fallout from Chernobyl. In Britain, Welsh, Cumbrian and Scottish sheep farmers have probably suffered more than anyone from that particular disaster, with loss of income and fears for their own families' health. It is estimated that several thousand Britons will eventually get cancer as a result of the radiation released from

Chernobyl, but as with almost all deaths resulting from radioactive contamination of the environment its victims will be anonymous.

INNOCENT UNTIL PROVEN GUILTY?

We are, however, at a disadvantage in an increasingly technological world, where political experts and scientists tell us what we should think about issues that intimately concern us. Most of the time scientists attempt to reassure us, telling us not to worry until something is proven guilty by lengthy tests or when the evidence in the environment is irrefutable. After all, most scientific research is paid for by government and industry.

We cannot see, touch or feel low level radiation, as we can some other modern hazards. If your family starts to itch when they put on clothes washed in biological detergent, you go back to the 'original formula', without needing any technical information at all – whereas you might eventually die from a cancer caused by radiation you were never aware of having been exposed to. Many modern dangers are difficult for the ordinary person to understand, and Thomas Kuhn, Harvard scientist and philosopher, has pointed out that one of the characteristics of modern scientific research is that it is no longer 'embodied in books addressed . . . to anyone who might be interested. . . . Instead, [it] will appear as brief articles addressed only to professional colleagues.'

Debates over the hole in the ozone layer and pollution in the North Sea have pointed out how supposedly scientific principles can be disastrous when applied to environmental problems. Scientists err on the side of caution, waiting until there is conclusive evidence of damage. When it comes to an ecosystem or an animal species, it may be far too late to save them. Instead, environmental advocates contend that we should apply precautionary principles: when damage is seen and there is a suspected link with human activity, the activity should be on trial. It should have to be proved safe before being used again. As E. F. Schumacher wrote in *Small is Beautiful*: 'Not that I wish in any way to belittle the evils of conventional air and water pollution; but we must recognise "dimensional differences" when we encounter them: radioactive pollution is an evil of an incomparably greater "dimension" than anything mankind has known before. One might even ask: what is the point of insisting on clean air, if the air is laden with radioactive particles? And even if the air could be protected, what is the point of it, if soil and water are being poisoned?'

TYPES OF RADIATION

Radiation is energy emitted as streams of particles or waves of vibrating electromagnetic energy. When these particles or vibrating energy strike matter, they set up corresponding vibrations which can be strong enough to disintegrate or permanently alter the matter. What makes radiation so important is that it does not simply kill individual cells but can alter DNA molecules and change the way cells reproduce. Ionizing radiation consists of alpha or beta particles, gamma rays, X-rays and part of the ultra-violet light spectrum. Radiation hazards and radiation discharges result from the decay of unstable atoms, some occurring naturally and some artificially produced in, for example, a nuclear reactor.

While nuclear or ionizing radiation consists of either particles or waves which can knock the electrons off other atoms (causing molecules to become 'ionized'), non-ionizing radiation consists only of energy waves and acts on matter by transferring energy, usually in the form of heat. Until recently it was thought to be harmless unless it produced heat, but there is much concern among scientists and the public about the health effects of the low levels of non-ionizing radiation found in all modern homes.

IONIZING RADIATION

When cells are affected by ionizing radiation, they generally die or fail to reproduce (in fact, radiation is sometimes used to kill cancerous cells), and a healthy body can destroy sick cells. Some damaged cells, may, however, reproduce abnormally, resulting in cancerous growth, and the damage can cause miscarriage or be transmitted as a genetic mutation. But the effects of cumulative, low-level radiation are hard to judge because it may be 40 years or more before we see the full effects of today's dose of radiation, and it is impossible to separate it clearly from other environmental influences on our health over that period of time.

In general, we only think of severe genetic defects and cancer deaths as the consequences of increased radiation in our environment, and the odds against this affecting any single person are, it is said, greater than dying in a car accident. Rosalie Bertell explains in *No Immediate Danger* that risk/benefit decision making balances 'health effects' (for you and me) against 'economic and social benefit' (this often turns out to be benefit for a particular industry or for national defence). These decisions require value judgements which misrepresent the equation, ignore long-term collective damage and often take no account of public opinion. In fact, the public has so little information to go on that most of us would be unable to make a reasoned decision.

Bertell claims that the 'early occurrence of heart disease, diabetes mellitus, arthritis, asthma or severe allergies – all resulting in a prolonged state of ill health' are part of the 'subtle widespread degradation of public health' which are never mentioned in official information about health risks from radiation.

Radiation is more hazardous to children than to adults, and most hazardous of all to unborn children, because body cells are dividing so rapidly – and because there is ultimately longer for cancer to develop. Although women are thought to be up to two-and-a-half times more vulnerable to radiation than men, genetic disorders can be passed on from either parent. Mild mutations can show themselves as allergies, asthma, hypertension, slight muscular or bone defects – which, says Bertell, 'leave the individual slightly less able to cope with ordinary stresses and hazards in the environment'. These genetic 'mistakes' are passed on from one generation to the next, made worse by increases in other hazardous elements of our modern environment (toxic chemicals, for example).

We are all exposed to some artificial radiation, at home and at work, because there are many sources of ionizing radiation in our environment. You may not be able to shut down Sellafield, but you can cut your exposure to radiation by making changes in the way you live. Increased awareness of the dangers of 'domestic' radiation will lead to a more determined attitude the next time you buy a house or go to the dentist – as well as the next time you vote.

As you read through the rest of this chapter, try to get an idea of the sources which apply to you and think about ways to reduce the total load. For example, someone exposed to radiation in the course of their work should try to reduce this occupational exposure while taking care to cut down on exposure from other sources.

SAFETY LEVELS

Any industry which has acknowledged environmental consequences and poses a risk to human health will talk of 'acceptable levels' and 'acceptable risk'. Unfortunately, researchers do not agree about acceptable risks. Estimating risk is difficult and determining the effects of various sorts of radiation is highly contentious. For every figure one expert presents another is thrown down to counter it. Statistics can tell us whether the rate of a particular disease in a given area is higher than average, but gives no clue as to causes. Besides this, results can be dramatically altered by simple adjustments in the boundary lines for a statistical survey. Researchers use different criteria and take different variables into account. In addition, risk estimates are based on cancer *deaths*, although this is not entirely satisfactory. Any cancer – even if completely curable – has important effects on your life, in terms of stress, finance, relationships and career.

There are no cumulative records on radiation exposure to members of the public from nuclear testing and the nuclear industry, which makes it virtually impossible to get a clear picture of the consequences of our defence and energy choices over the past 40 or 50 years. None the less, worker studies show that standards have been set for toxic substances for which there are no safe levels and there is no safe level for exposure to ionizing radiation.

The permissible radiation doses for both public and workers were set in 1957 by the International Commission on Radiological Protection (ICRP), an organization that has strong links with nuclear industry (and which, by the way, has never appointed a female member). The standards were based on then-current research into the effects of the atomic bombs dropped on Japan in 1945, and although recent research has shown that these effects were greatly underestimated, the levels have not been changed, in spite of international pressure on the ICRP.

A number of environmental groups and trade unions are calling for an immediate reduction in permissible levels by a factor of 5, aiming for an eventual reduction by a factor of 10. The present levels are set at 5 milliSieverts (mSv) per annum for members of the public and 50 mSv for nuclear employees. The UK's National Radiological Protection Board (NRPB) has recommended cutting public exposure to a maximum of 1 mSv ($^1/_5$ of the current level) and worker exposure to 15 mSv ($^1/_3$ of the current level). These recommendations are not, however, legally enforceable and the idea that acceptable radiation doses for employees should be ten times higher than for the rest of us is questionable.

BACKGROUND RADIATION AND RADON

Light, radium, radon, uranium and potassium in the earth are natural sources of ionizing radiation. Living at high elevation, and travelling in an aeroplane, exposes people to radiation from cosmic rays. These have always been part of the environment human beings have lived in, but the term 'background' radiation is not quite as straightforward as we are led to believe. It includes naturally occurring radiation, but also covers fallout from nuclear weapons testing over the past half century and artificial radiation from fission products after they have been in the environment for a year. 'Background' radiation levels have steadily risen over the past 50 years, giving a deceptive turn to any statistics on radiation from the nuclear industry. This is an extraordinary state of affairs – do we consider extremely persistent and dangerous chemicals like PCBs part of the natural composition of sea water simply because they have been there for some time?

■Radiation At Home

The form in which natural radiation affects us at home is as radon, a colourless and odourless gas given off by the radioactive decay of elements in the earth. The degree to which radon is a hazard depends a great deal on where you live and on what your home is built of. In the British Isles, trouble spots include Cornwall, Devon and Glasgow (where radon seeps from the radon-bearing granite many houses are built from). In well-insulated, poorly ventilated buildings radiation has been known to reach a level of twice the legal limit set for nuclear power workers, and an estimated 100,000 homes in the UK are affected. In the US, a recent report suggests that 20 per cent of homes may be affected by radon.

An annual 1600 cases of lung cancer in the UK have been attributed to radon and it is the usual cause of lung cancer in non-smokers. A public health warning in the US compares the radon levels in many homes to smoking a half pack of cigarettes a day. Polonium-210, an alpha emitter like radon and its daughter products, is also found in tobacco smoke.

Government agencies seem happier to talk about the dangers of radon than about other radiation hazards, because it can be treated as separate from the nuclear industry. However, some of the radioactive products which produce radon have been removed from their relatively harmless natural state – by being 'blasted out of the ground with dynamite or leached with acids, and pulverised into very small particles' – in order to provide material for nuclear power stations or atomic weapons and are hardly what most of us would call 'natural' radiation.

Glass, ceramics, bricks, cement, natural gas, phosphate fertilizers, gypsum board and even deep well water can release small quantities of radon, depending on where they come from. As radon problems increase, more care will have to be taken with the materials used in building, as well as with where we build, and how homes are ventilated and insulated.

The real issue is stopping radon entering the house through the floor in the first place. General rules for homes with high radon levels are:

1. floors and walls should be sealed with caulking and cement.

2. good ventilation is crucial, especially on the ground floor; and

3. basements can be separately ventilated with a small exhaust fan and stairs can be sealed with a weatherstripped door.

For radon testing and advice, see Sources.

■Medical Radiation

Medical diagnosis by X-ray is the largest source of artificial radiation that affects humans. On average we receive higher organ doses from medical procedures (which include X-rays, radiation treatment and radioactive drugs) than from any other source except rare industrial accidents.

Medical X-rays are estimated to cause between 350 and 2000 extra cancers per year in the UK, half of them fatal, as well as some 600 serious genetic disorders in babies. It is impossible to determine accurately the number of minor genetic disorders and health problems they cause.

In spite of these facts, most people have no idea that they could be adversely affected by X-ray treatment. Only pregnant women are advised to avoid unnecessary X-rays (in the past, however, these were used for routine monitoring during pregnancy, as ultrasound is today). If it is unsafe to X-ray foetuses, what about X-raying the ovaries, which contain the eggs that will produce future offspring? And if we don't know, shouldn't we be erring on the side of caution?

Of course the benefits of X-rays frequently outweigh the risks involved. If your leg has been shattered in an accident, you are unlikely to quibble about the X-rays needed to make a decision about how to set it. The important point about this, however, is that even when an X-ray is essential the doses given by different equipment, in different hospitals, can vary by as much as a factor of 1000. It's crucial that we ask questions and make a fuss about this all too routine exposure to radiation. Be a pain – it's your DNA.

Dental X-rays are another source of radiation exposure. Although the British Dental Association takes no official position on how often routine X-rays should be done, some US recommendations are for routine dental X-rays no more often than every 5–10 years. A full mouth X-ray can be the equivalent of 18 partial shots, and is something to be particularly wary of.

■X-ray checklist

1. Avoid precautionary and routine medical and dental X-rays.

2. Discuss alternative diagnosis methods with your practitioner. If a doctor suggests high radiation X-rays, insist on discussing the situation to your complete satisfaction before going ahead.

3. Women in childbearing years should have X-rays only in the ten days following menstruation. (This so-called 'ten day rule' has been officially abandoned.)

4. No X-rays during pregnancy or while trying to conceive, unless absolutely unavoidable.

5. No X-rays for children unless genuine medical emergency.

6. Insist that X-ray films are transferred with you if you are referred to another doctor.

7. Tell your doctor that you want to limit X-rays to a minimum, and ask for an explanation and dose estimate before agreeing to any X-ray treatment.

8. Do not agree to 'defensive' X-rays (a problem in litigious America, where doctors like to document every step of treatment – and a growing problem in the UK).

9. Ask the radiologist what dose you are getting and do not accept 'very small' as an answer.

10. Ensure that you are wearing a lead shield to protect the rest of your body, especially sex organs any time you are X-rayed (even at the dentist).

11. If possible, choose a radiologist or hospital with efficient, modern equipment (which can achieve the same results with far lower X-ray doses).

■ Consumer Products

There is no legislation in the UK governing radioactive materials in products – from luminous dials, anti-static devices and smoke detectors, to camera lenses and ceramic tiles, enamelled badges and glow-in-the-dark toys – we use every day. In most cases, doses are very small, and it is impossible to compute an average dose for the entire population. But the misuse of some items, particularly smoke detectors, can lead to higher exposure levels, and there is an inevitable problem with disposal and contamination of manufacturing sites.

The nuclear industry provides a cheap source of Americium-241, an ionizing radiation source which is used in smoke detectors. What could look more innocuous than that white plastic disc on the ceiling? They are sold without any sort of warning on the package or on the detector, but there is an increase in radiation around them for up to 10 cm.

Optical smoke detectors work for smouldering fires, but the common ionization chamber model is required for the flash fires which have become a hazard with the advent of highly combustible foam materials in furniture. The ionizing material is not well protected and a child could prise the detector apart.

The NRPB can test and approve products, but have to charge for the service. There is no legal requirement for manufacturers to have their goods tested, however, and consumers are for the most part unaware of the danger. Some environmental radiation researchers believe that consumer goods with a health or safety purpose should be able to use radioactive materials only if there is no alternative, and only then under strict controls, and that there is no justification for using these materials in other consumer goods.

THE NUCLEAR INDUSTRY

The problems and risks of nuclear radiation are the last things many of us want to think about, because there seems so little we can do about it. Things aren't really quite so bad as that, fortunately. Although we have been told for years that nuclear power is our only hope for the future, public resistance has been growing, and economic pressures (including the largely unknown, but politically astronomic, costs of decommissioning power stations) are making it look less and less likely to expand as planned. The industry's continuing insistence that all is well – in spite of the evidence – is beginning to look almost touchingly naïve.

Nuclear fuel and weaponry pose risks to human beings in a variety of ways. Mining and manufacture, reactor operation, fuel reprocessing, plutonium storage and waste, and fallout from nuclear testing. Indigenous populations have suffered most, both from uranium mining (in the US and Canada, Australia and Africa) and from weapons testing (particularly in the South Pacific).

The security threat from reprocessing nuclear waste was discussed in Chapter 7, but another consideration is routine and occasional emissions from nuclear power stations. Britain has specialized in reprocessing nuclear waste, from other countries as well as its own; in 1994 British officials were discussing plans to reprocess and possibly store US nuclear waste, although this contravened international agreements that industrialized countries should deal with their own toxic waste. Sellafield, formerly Windscale, is thought to be responsible for over half the worldwide radioactive emissions from power stations, according to the Oxford Political Ecology Research Group. There are higher than normal environmental levels of radiation in seawater around most of Britain's coastline.

The problem and eventual cost of nuclear waste storage cannot be underestimated. There is a misleading linguistic ploy being used, contrasting deep sea 'disposal' with other forms of 'storage'. The fact is that the *only* choice with nuclear waste is storage, in deep repositories, shallow dumps or repackaged for permanent storage at nuclear stations. The issue of environmental justice raises its head, as the industry looks for acceptable sites for storage in areas where there are either few people or few people with political clout.

At present, the quantities of nuclear waste already generated have already reached alarming proportions without any acceptable storage option being found. It seems incredible that nuclear power has been allowed to expand for decades, while the experts tried half-heartedly to figure out a way of dealing with the inevitable and highly dangerous waste products.

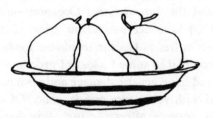

FOOD IRRADIATION

Food irradiation is legal in Britain, but it seems unlikely to be much used because of intense public resistance. I find this an encouraging sign, a technology rejected because people are not convinced that it performs a needed task and because they are uncomfortable about potential risks, as well as about its links to the nuclear power industry. Irradiation is, however, being used in other countries and we shouldn't assume that it will not become a major issue again.

The beneficiaries of irradiation are the nuclear industry and certain segments of the food industry. Irradiation would make it possible for manufacturers to sell lower quality food which would last longer in commercial storage or on the supermarket shelf, and still appear fresh and wholesome. Spices from India *have* to be irradiated; otherwise they would be full of weavils. Contaminated and spoiled food can be sterilized, and some forms of contamination can even be disguised through the use of irradiation. Early research into food irradiation took place as part of the 'Atoms for Peace' programme, so the technique was developed by the US Army, not by the food industry, and the preferred isotopes which are used to irradiate food are products of nuclear reactors. Irradiation has been aptly described as 'a technology looking for a use'.

Rather than eliminate the need for additives in food, irradiation would require a new range of additives to deal with the effects of irradiation. For example, polyphosphates would be necessary to reduce the bleeding of meats and antioxidants to offset the rancid flavours which can develop after irradiation. There is some evidence that toxins and viruses can mutate as a result of irradiation, and the International Organization of Consumer Unions (IOCU) is concerned about trials that have shown increased levels of free radicals in irradiated food. Although free radicals are essential to some biological processes, they can also harm cells, producing genetic damage and even cancer, and they are associated with premature ageing. The IOCU is also concerned about adverse effects – including lowered immune response, birth rates, and sperm counts and blood clotting, and increased kidney damage and tumours – found in studies of animals fed irradiated food. No adequate testing has been done on how irradiation acts on the many food additives in common use.

One industry claim has been that the technique would cut down on food poisoning, but if chicken is irradiated to kill dangerous salmonella bacteria, the technique would also kill organisms which are natural competitors of botulinum (a bacterium which causes a lethal form of food poisoning) and organisms which would naturally cause a putrid odour (which tells us that something is not safe to eat), but would not destroy the deadly botulinus toxin itself.

Irradiated food is not radioactive, but employees in irradiation plants are exposed to the same health risks as other radiation workers. We need to ask whether we would want to buy products which carry this 'cost' in risk to human health. Irradiation plants would add to the amount of radioactive emissions into the environment, and to our radioactive waste 'storage problem'.

There is presently no certain means of detecting irradiated foodstuffs, which makes any idea of regulating the labelling of irradiated food impossible. The industry has come up with some amusing suggestions for irradiation symbols, none of which include the word 'irradiated'. In the US a graphic depicting a flower is used. Consumer advocates are insistent that irradiated food must be clearly labelled as such so shoppers have a choice, but no legislation has been devised to cover prepared foods containing irradiated ingredients.

MICROWAVES, TELEVISION AND RADAR

We are surrounded by electrical appliances which have potentially serious effects on our well-being. Think of the electrical equipment in your home, the power cables above your head or running underground along the streets, as well as the TV and radio broadcasting networks which have become an essential part of our lives. Although most of us have a vague notion that leaking microwave ovens are a risky business and that we shouldn't sit too near the TV, the real dangers of these forms of radiation are largely uncertain.

Civilian and military radar technicians, microwave workers, TV, radio and other communication personnel are exposed to microwave radiation. So are the rest of us, from TV and radio broadcasting stations and radar systems. FM towers pose a particular hazard because the radiation they emit is 'pulsed'.

Microwave cataracts are a well-documented health hazard to workers, but microwave radiation also seems to cause a variety of non-thermal effects. Tests with animals have shown an almost immediate decline in work performance and decision-making capacity, along with chronic stress problems, inefficiency and central nervous system disturbance. Headaches and nausea are other observed reactions, and microwave radiation is suspected of causing cancer and genetic damage. In one case, the children of men who worked as radar technicians at a military base in Alabama in the US had an exceptionally high rate of birth defects.

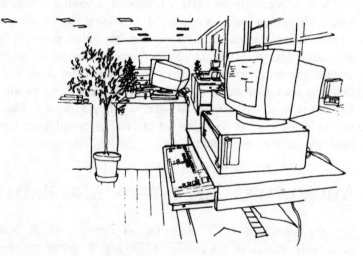

VIDEO DISPLAY UNITS (VDUs)

There has been a considerable amount of publicity about the dangers of VDUs. These are computer monitors or screens, and workers who spend most of their time in front of them have been found to suffer from a variety of ailments, ranging from headaches, eye strain, fatigue, anxiety and depression, to repetitive strain injury (RSI). Even more serious is the suspected connection with reproductive problems.

Attention was first drawn to this when a group of women working on VDUs at the *Toronto Star*, in Canada, had an unusu-

ally high rate of miscarriage. Other studies have confirmed that
there is a higher rate of miscarriage among VDU workers, as well
as a higher rate of birth defects. The extent of the risk, and the
exact reasons for it, are unclear. Most VDUs do not emit more
than very low levels of ionizing radiation (what most of us think
of when we hear the word 'radiation'). They do give out varying
amount of VLF (very low frequency) and ELF (extremely low
frequency) electromagnetic waves, and these are suspected of
causing the problems.

Some companies have policies that workers who use VDUs for
more than 26 hours a week must have a 15-minute break every 3
hours. It also helps to have mobile keyboards, anti-glare screens
and offices with diffuse overhead lighting. These regulations are,
in fact, minimal and far more stringent safety measures will eventually need to be taken. The VDU Workers' Rights Campaign
suggest that no employee should spend more than four hours or
half the working day at a VDU, that they should take regular
breaks and that computers should be properly shielded.

■What You Can Do To Your Home Computer

You can purchase anti-glare screens that also shield the user from
radiation. This shielding also eliminates the problem of static.
Many computer users know to their chagrin how static can wipe
out a day's work in a flash and it can result in invisible paper dust
in the air bombarding the VDU worker in the face, contributing
to eye and skin problems. It also helps to avoid synthetic carpets
and other materials in your computer room, and improved
humidity will lessen static. Plants improve air quality and humidity, and you can spray water into the air or on your skin (scent it
with a little lavender oil). Keep the central heating as low as possible. Many people find that ionizers improve the atmosphere
too.

ELECTROMAGNETIC RADIATION

The effects of low-level electromagnetic radiation have been of
concern to a number of biologists for many years but only

recently have they attracted much public attention. One study showed a 40 per cent increase in suicide rate among people living under high voltage power lines, and low levels of electromagnetic radiation seem to cause depression and mood changes. In Britain, public concern is increasing. The Electricity Association funds an Electromagnetic Field (EMF) unit and the National Radiological Protection Board is being forced to study the effects of low-level radiation.

Electromagnetic radiation is not all bad. The earth has its own magnetic fields, which govern such things as animals' migration patterns, and human tissue has electric and electromagnetic properties. These fields are sometimes used to promote the healing of broken bones and wounds, and Russian research suggests that the difference between living and non-living matter is electricity. Western medicine is based on a biochemical understanding of the body and its systems, ignoring the likelihood that electrical influences are equally important in growth, healing and metabolism. During the twentieth century, intense and chaotic electromagnetic phenomena – some call it electromagnetic pollution – have become common throughout much of the world.

Although the most worrying effects have been noted under high-voltage power lines, all of us are surrounded by this form of artificial radiation in our homes, from mains currents, electricity meters and burglar alarms, to clock radios, cookers and irons. Health effects include childhood leukaemia, higher rates of miscarriage, increased allergies, brain tumours and breast cancer. Several recent US studies have shown higher cancer rates in people exposed to strong electromagnetic fields, and a study in New Zealand found an excess of leukaemia among electronic equipment assemblers, and radio and television repairmen. One US research team found high levels of electromagnetic radiation in some surprising places: near a dishwasher and in a café with faulty wiring. Chemists are concerned that exposure to magnetic fields increases the body's production of free radicals, causing harmful chain reactions which damage the immune system.

Electromagnetic radiation in our homes may well prove to be a significant hazard, and is likely to be difficult to reduce, given our dependence on electricity and electrical appliances. Until we know more, sensible precautions include the following.

▶ Sit as far as possible from VDUs and televisions, and minimize the time you spend in front of them.

▶ Use a radiation shield on an old CRT monitor or buy a VDU that has passed Swedish radiation standards.

▶ Choose hand-operated appliances whenever possible.

▶ Unplug appliances when not in use (they continue to produce magnetic fields even if switched off).

▶ Reduce the amount of electrical equipment in bedrooms and children's playrooms.

▶ Use a hot water bottle to warm your bed instead of an electric blanket.

▶ Move beds at least 4 ft from electric night storage heaters, clock radios, electricity meters, transformers and burglar alarms.

▶ Read microwave oven instructions carefully and keep seals clean.

▶ Cook with gas rather than a microwave.

▶ Ask your electricity company to check magnetic fields in and around your home. Many will do this for no charge. They can replace cabling with modern, low-emission products.

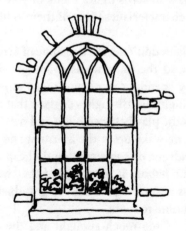

14

LIGHT

They say Native Americans danced for rain. In Britain, many people would do a dance if they thought it would bring sunshine at the weekend. We need sunlight and love it. It affects how we feel, how we spend our time and even where we live. Good designers know human beings are 'phototropic' – that is, they naturally gravitate towards light. Think of your favourite rooms. What are their characteristics? One of them is likely to be diffuse natural light.

The British Isles don't get the sunshine of Greece or Australia, but we compound the natural disadvantages of dull skies and dark winters by spending more and more of our time indoors, under artificial lighting. Biologists suggest that our 'biorhythms' may depend on the play between night and day. This seems obvious – after all, we wake up in the morning and go to sleep after dark. But the advent of convenient and cheap artificial lighting has changed our habits. It is estimated that we receive at least one-quarter less natural light than our grandparents because we spend so much time indoors.

The dangers of too much sunlight and the ageing effects of excessive tanning are much in the news. But moderation is crucial. Modern living tends to isolate us from direct sunlight: we spend a lot of time behind glass, either windows or spectacles. Even when the sun does shine we don't get the full benefit of natural light. Light can promote health, and a lack of it contributes to depressive disorders in some people.

THE OZONE LAYER

The most alarming environmental aspect of light is the danger posed by the destruction of the ozone layer, which acts as a buffer between us and highly dangerous ultraviolet (UV) radiation from the sun. The hole in the ozone layer over the Antarctic was no surprise to environmentalists who had been predicting the breakdown of the ozone for some 15 years. The tragedy is that whatever we do has come much later than it might have, and too late to prevent considerable ecological damage and many cases of cancer.

Ozone is a volatile gas with molecules consisting of three oxygen atoms. It forms an essential protective layer around the earth and happens to be vulnerable to a number of gases, particularly those containing chlorine, which are manufactured and released by humankind. (Ozone is a pollutant at ground level and contributes to smog in hot weather.) Chlorofluorocarbons, or CFCs, are a group of chemicals mainly used as the propellant in aerosol cans (deodorants, hairsprays, furniture polish, insecticide etc.), as well as in the 'blowing' of polystyrene packaging and in refrigerants (the liquids which circulate in refrigerators and freezers to carry heat away).

According to Friends of the Earth we can expect to see a sharp rise in the number of skin cancers, as well as an increase in eye diseases like cataracts and damage to agricultural crops (will they have to be sprayed with sunscreen?). Even if all CFC production was stopped now, there are hundreds of thousands of tons of CFCs hanging over our heads and the effects of a damaged ozone layer will be with us for at least 100 years.

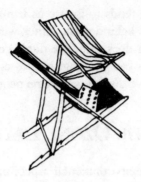

DANGEROUS LIGHT

It is tempting to strip all one's clothes off and bask for as many heedless hours as possible when the opportunity presents itself, but this is a luxury no one can afford, given the dangers of excessive sunbathing. It's hard to be sensible, knowing that we get so much less sun than people in other countries, but we have all the more reason today to take warnings about sunbathing seriously. People of Celtic descent have a high skin cancer rate; there is even a risk scale called 'celticity'! An EU cancer map shows that the rate of malignant melanoma, a fatal skin cancer, is high in parts of England, Wales and Ireland (much higher than in France, but lower than Germany and Denmark). Many Britons have fair, sun-sensitive skin and even Britons with darker skins need sun protection, as the thinning of the ozone layer allows more dangerous UV radiation to reach us.

But if you can't resist the temptation to tan, at least moderate your goal to a pleasant golden shade and give your skin plenty of time to achieve it. Every chemist now stocks a wide range of sun-blocking creams, numbered on a scale from 1 to at least 20. The lower numbers are for darker skin or faster tanning, and 20 is a complete block. But put it on before you go out. And all creams need to be reapplied frequently if you are swimming, or sweating. Start with as little as two minutes on each side and gradually increase your daily dose of direct sunlight, but never so much that you find your skin slightly reddened afterwards.

Sun beds have been heavily promoted as safer than tanning outside, but much of the information consumers receive is misleading. Shorter UV-B rays have received bad publicity because they cause superficial reddening and burning, while longer UV-A rays have been advertised as safe 'tanning' rays because they develop melanin particles in the skin and create a tan without burning. Recent research shows that UV-A rays are probably more damaging in the long run than UV-B 'burning' rays because they cause premature and irreversible ageing of the skin, just as the sun does.

TIPS ON SAFE EXPOSURE TO SUNLIGHT

* Wear a moisturizer with sunblock in it all the time. This will become more important as time passes, especially as you get older.
* Shop around to find an alternative if your skin reacts badly to PABA, a common sunblock ingredient.
* If you have one, cherish an English rose complexion and aim to be fashionably pale. It's absolutely true that Englishwomen (and men) have better skin than their American cousins, who suffer from too much sun, extremes of climate, and centrally heated and air-conditioned buildings.
* Spend time outside, but not in direct sunlight.
* Beware reflected light and cloudy days – as much as 80 per cent of the sun's radiation makes it through the clouds.
* Consider wearing sunglasses if you are in the sun a great deal, to avoid eye problems later in life.
* Make sure the lenses absorb 100 per cent of both UV-A and UV-B light.
* Sunbathe cautiously, if at all, particularly if you have fair skin.
* Stay away from sun beds.

- If you must have brown legs, use a self-tan lotion.
- Examine yourself for skin growths, itchy patches, sores that won't heal, changes in moles or coloured areas. These could be cancerous and can almost always be treated successfully if caught early.
- Contribute to Friends of the Earth, who have been campaigning to save the ozone layer for years.

LIGHT AND HEALTH

Sunlight has exciting effects on our metabolic rate and hormones, and too much darkness can lead to low spirits and depression. A few people suffer from a condition called seasonal affective disorder (SAD) during dark winter months. Characteristic symptoms are severe winter depression, unrelated to other events in one's life, which lifts at the arrival of spring, accompanied by cravings for carbohydrates, weight gain and excessive sleeping.

While some people suffer from SAD so severely that they need specialist treatment, most of us are familiar with winter blues. Our Christmas celebrations, full of colour and sound and light, sensibly fall at the winter solstice, when days are shortest. It seems reasonable to assume that we also need a little help during the darkest months of the year, whether from special full-spectrum lighting indoors or an effort to spend time outside.

Dr Alfred Lewy, an expert on light and circadian rhythms, has found that properly timed exposure to bright light will reset your body clock after a long flight. For example, when returning to the UK from New York, morning light will reduce jet lag.

Light improves our health in other ways. It used to be our primary source of vitamin D, formed by the sun in the oils on our skin and then absorbed by the body. Today, we generally need supplements or foods 'fortified' with vitamin D because we don't get enough from natural sources, and soap and frequent bathing washes most of what we get directly from the sun straight down the drain. Lack of vitamin D can lead to poor calcium absorption and in turn to osteoporosis in elderly people.

Before trying to improve your indoor lighting, think about how to get more direct sunlight.

▶ Spend as much time as you can outside. Catch a bus 15 minutes' walk down the road or go for a walk at lunch time.

▶ Choose outdoor activities in preference to indoor ones: tennis instead of squash; running rather than a rowing machine.

▶ Walk or cycle instead of driving.

▶ Keep track of how much time you spend in real light each day and how you feel as a result. An absolute minimum is 15 minutes in summer and 30 minutes in winter (when the sun is less intense), but try to get much more than that.

▶ Try to work close to a window, preferably with it open.

▶ Make a sunny part of your garden an outdoor room by equipping it with a table, comfortable chairs and adequate protection from direct summer sun. Informal and permanent seats, even if only a low brick wall, make a garden far more hospitable.

▶ If you live in a flat, it may be possible to turn the area near a window or a narrow balcony into a sunny spot to work and eat.

▶ Check the light levels around your home. A camera with a light sensor in the viewfinder is a surprising tool – a room can be considerably duller than you think.

▶ Increase light levels inside.

▶ Experiment with different types of artificial lighting to see what you feel best with.

▶ Do your eyes a favour by emphasizing any views you have available: one of the problems with urban living is that we seldom have to look at anything further away than a retreating bus. Or go for walks in the country at weekends, where you can use your eyes. Try counting sheep on a distant hillside.

▶ Don't wear sunglasses permanently. They are useful when there is excessive glare and do prevent eye damage if you are in the sun a great deal, but because they filter out specific wavebands of light they can contribute to light deprivation. We need some sunlight unfiltered by lenses or window panes.

LIGHT AND THE ENVIRONMENT

There are conflicts between the environment and human health that require additional research. In fact, the only perfect environmental solution would be to use sunlight for lighting and nothing else. Even with solar-powered lighting there are manufacturing and disposal issues to consider, though these systems are the best option and perfectly feasible in sunny parts of the world. In Britain we will continue to rely on artificial lighting much of the time, and what we need is the ability to make best possible use of natural light when it is available, together with the most efficient and healthy artificial lighting we can find.

■Fluorescent Lights

Many people who have lived or worked under fluorescent lighting are instinctively aware of how uncomfortable it is, though we don't know quite why. Fluorescent lighting is standard in offices, banks and shops because it is cheaper to run than incandescent, needing only one-quarter of the energy in continuous use. It saves energy, though there are polluting chemicals used in manufacturing various types of bulbs.

Recent studies show that improving the quality of light at work reduces absenteeism, cuts down on headaches, eyestrain and fatigue. Even though we are not consciously aware of the 100-times-a-second flicker of fluorescent lights (except with a dud bulb and we all know how irritating that is), on a subconscious level it is extremely stressful. New types of fluorescent lights flicker much faster than the old ones – at up to 30,000 times a minute – and are much easier on both eye and brain.

At home, you can fit full-spectrum bulbs in fluorescent fixtures, but at the office the best option is mixed lighting sources, with adjustable lights at each work station. You may be able to use an incandescent desk lamp and turn off the overhead fluorescent lights. If not – and many workers have no choice about the continuous overhead fluorescent lighting – you might mention the new type of bulb to the relevant person, and the recent work done by the Applied Psychology Unit at Cambridge University about increased efficiency with better lighting.

■Full-Spectrum Lights

There is agreement about at least one of the problems of artificial lighting. The spectrum of light produced by artificial sources is different from natural daylight. Daylight has a more even spread of light across the coloured wave bands, with a higher proportion of blue and green. Make-up artists know how much of a difference the colour of light makes.

When I asked a lighting consultant which type of light he preferred he said promptly, 'Halogen, it makes things look wonderful. You should see jewellery under it.' 'What about people's faces?' I asked. 'Oh,' he said and sighed. 'Faces. Well, faces are difficult. Candlelight is good.'

You know the problem of buying a tie to go with a particular suit and finding that it is a different colour when you get it home? You are advised to 'check the colour in daylight', but in a big department store this is virtually impossible. Some people need to see colours accurately for their work, while at home cooking is easier and pleasanter under natural or full-spectrum lighting, as is looking at yourself in the mirror first thing in the morning.

Full spectrum bulbs are not always easy to find. See Sources for a mail order supplier. A complete set of full spectrum lights for treating SAD is expensive and includes a special treatment case, but individual tubes can be installed in ordinary fluorescent fittings from the DIY shop.

HOME DESIGN AND ORIENTATION

The solution to the apparent conflict with human health needs for sufficient natural, full spectrum light and the environmentalists' contention that we should use energy-saving fluorescent bulbs is to use artificial lighting more carefully and increase the amount of natural light we use in our homes and offices. Modern buildings are designed on the principle that artificial lighting is just as good as, perhaps better than, natural daylight and architects of the past don't seem to have given a great deal of consideration to the provision of light in houses. Because poorly insulated windows let vast amounts of heat out, old farmhouses tended to be built with thick walls and small windows.

Here are some design principles to keep in mind when you arrange rooms and lighting. In addition to improving the light quality indoors, you'll reduce energy consumption too.

▶ Choose, if you can, a southerly exposure for house and garden. Because we live in the northern hemisphere, the sun is always in the southern part of the sky.

▶ Consider the times rooms are used. Your kitchen is probably used most in the late afternoon and early evening, but it's also nice to have a bright kitchen in the morning. Bedrooms need light in the morning and sitting rooms in the evening. Playrooms and rooms used as office or study probably need as much light as possible throughout the day. Formal sitting and dining rooms are often used only in the evening, and can sometimes be switched to a less light-valuable part of the house.

▶ Arrange rooms by the availability and timing of daylight. Rooms you use in the morning should face east, rooms which are used in the afternoon and evening should face west.

▶ Look outside, at anything which gets in the way of the light which reaches you. There isn't much to be done about the house across the street or a railway station, but trees and shrubs can be pruned or even moved. If the problem is acute, remove them and plant replacements somewhere else.

▶ Dark rooms, facing north or a blank brick wall, or with no windows at all, should be used least.

▶ Even in Britain we can get too much light, which makes a room hot and full of glare. If you have a room in which you could bake fish on a July afternoon, take this into account when deciding on layout. But it is much easier to block some of the light than it is to maximize light during dark months. Curtains and blinds can be used (an outside blind is most effective), and eaves and deciduous trees can be used to block hot summer sun, while allowing low winter sun to enter the house. Another appealing long-term solution is to grow climbing plants around the windows. Choose varieties which lose their leaves in winter so they don't block light when it is in short supply. In the short term, try morning glories and other annual climbers.

▶ Skylights are excellent for illuminating hallways and stairs. If you are making alterations in your house, think about placing small windows to maximize lighting where it is most needed.

▶ If you are buying or building a new house, a long east–west axis has been shown to minimize energy consumption by keeping the heat in during the winter and out during the summer.

▶ Increase indoor light by placing cheap, fixed windows in interior walls and by using glazed doors between rooms when privacy is not important. Both can have curtains to pull if necessary.

▶ Use mirrors freely, as if they were pictures to hang on the wall. This can be very cheap, and very pretty. I like old mirrors, the kind you can find in junk shops for a couple of pounds. The glass is bevelled, and there is something about the silvering (perhaps with a few dark spots) and the slight irregularities in the glass which makes the light they reflect prettier than new mirror glass. Mirrors can be framed, too; old frames can be picked up cheaply – try house clearance places or auctions. Have old mirrors cut by a specialist firm (look under 'Mirrors – Antique' in the Yellow Pages). Try a long mirror between windows. The Chinese system of design, *feng shui*, suggests that mirrors and other reflective objects create a serene atmosphere and encourage more harmonious and flowing movements.

▶ Create a view. A friend of mine has a small-paned window (salvaged from a demolition site) hanging in her rather dingy hall. It has delicate lace curtains tied back with ribbons, and behind the glass is a print of a country landscape. The innocent trompe-l'oeil gives a feeling of spaciousness. This technique could be really useful in a windowless bathroom and you could use a mirror instead of a print. At Brown's Hotel in London there is a stained glass window set into an internal wall, lit from behind and heavily draped to match the other windows. The impression is one of windows on both sides of the room – very pleasant on a wet January afternoon while sipping tea and eating cucumber sandwiches!

WINDOW DRESSING

- To maximize available light, curtains should pull entirely off the window, which means a longer track or rail. Simple tiebacks can make a difference.
- Make sure that blinds are easy to pull all the way up, out of the way. Curtains and blinds should be easy to draw.
- Shutters are efficient insulators and pull well off windows during the day.
- Windows should open wide. Window glass blocks the beneficial rays from sunlight, but with windows which open on nice days you can have fresh air and sunshine inside. Casement windows and floor-to-ceiling French windows are terrific.
- A window seat, or a low sill with a chair nearby, makes a pleasant sunny spot for you, and for the cat.
- Burglar alarms can be a disincentive to opening windows because you have to ensure that they are all closed again properly to reset the alarm. Try to choose a system that doesn't present this problem.
- Clean windows let in more light – good window cleaners are worth their weight in gold. Skylights need to be cleaned regularly. Lightbulbs also need to be cleaned with a slightly damp cloth when the bulb is cold. Lampshades gradually darken with dust, so brush or vacuum them occasionally to let more light shine through.
- If privacy is a problem, let plants climb around a window (try something rambling and easy to grow like jasmine, or climbing roses – both will bring in wafts of scent when in bloom). Ivy and other climbers will grow happily in tubs or windowboxes.

15

CREATING
A GARDEN

Gardening is an important part of the Green Home, whether you garden on 5 acres in Herefordshire or in a windowbox four storeys up in south London. Growing food is a fundamental part of human life. How can we appreciate the food we eat, and take proper care in buying and preparing it, if it always comes off supermarket shelves? Producing at least a little of our own food provides an immediate connection with natural life cycles. Growing things is good for you (fresh air, sunshine and exercise) and home grown food is good for you (delicious, nutritious and uncontaminated by artificial chemicals). Even if you stick to growing non-edible shrubs and flowers, they disguise unattractive features, offer privacy, shelter and food for wildlife, and generally beautify our surroundings.

City dwellers don't have much space, tall buildings shade what little ground they have, gardens are built on heaps of builders' rubble and getting hold of manure is virtually impossible, but it is city dwellers who have the most to gain from even a tiny garden. You may have nothing but a small patio, or tiny portion of shared garden, or a balcony, or a rooftop. These all present exciting challenges! You have the great advantage that everyone will rave about the transformation, no matter what you do, and the special pleasure of creating something from nothing.

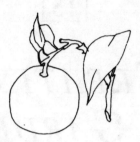

GREEN GARDENING

The following green gardening checklist will give you an idea of the basic points to be aware of:

▶ organic growing techniques;
▶ native varieties;
▶ permanent rather than disposable plantings;
▶ self-sowing annuals;
▶ spaced paving rather than concrete;
▶ wildlife corners;
▶ natural materials.

■ Getting Started

Before you start a gardening project, assess your circumstances. How much ground do you have (if you have any at all)? Is it sunny or shady? Boggy or dry? What about other space to grow on: walls, patios, steps? Indoors, is there enough light to grow plants? (Don't give up – growlights will transform even a sunless dungeon.) If you have a conservatory or a balcony your choices expand considerably.

Just as important, how much time do you have? Who will share the work? If you are away a lot, is there someone to take over the watering? And how much money do you have to spend? If you have a largish garden and don't seem to manage to keep up with it, consider paying a student to help with the heavy work. A well-kept garden will entice you to use it more, and muscle often costs less than expensive fertilizers and expensive plants which die because they've gone into the wrong spot or are never watered. A large garden could also be profitably shared with someone who wants space for a vegetable garden – you could exchange a patch for a share of the produce or for some help in the rest of the garden.

And how much do you know about gardening? The worst problem for most of us is that we didn't grow up helping our parents maintain a garden or grow vegetables. Green thumbs can be cultivated, and depend on a combination of knowledge, instinct and keen observation. The gardener becomes attuned to rhythms and signals which other people miss, and perhaps for this reason many people suffering from stress find gardening a particularly satisfying pastime.

■Bulbs

One fun way to start gardening is by growing bulbs to bloom during the winter or even for Christmas if you plant at the right time. They can be planted in bulb fibre, but grow better in either commercial potting compost or garden soil. After flowering, find a spot for them in the garden. Hyacinths, huge heavy stalks of blossom the first year, will gradually get smaller until eventually they look like large bluebells. You'll need to buy new bulbs each year for indoor potting.

Unfortunately, some bulbs on sale in Britain have come from the wild, principally cyclamen dug on Turkish hillsides. The EC is considering a control on their import, but at present up to 2.4 million of these wild bulbs are sold in Europe each year. Brian Matthews of Kew Gardens says that because the bulbs are generally packed in Holland there is no definite way to identify them, but if you are buying cyclamen watch out for misshapen and irregularly-sized tubers, signs that they are likely to have come from the wild.

■Garbage Gardening

Another way to start gardening without too much commitment is to buy a bag of potting compost – or use some (sifted) garden soil – and fill a couple of pots or cottage cheese tubs with a hole punched in the bottom for drainage. Put them in a sunny spot, if you have one, out of draughts.

Then start collecting seeds. Orange and lemon pips grow nicely, and will turn into attractive little trees (even in a dark corner they seem to stay dark green and healthy – although you won't get fruit, the leaves are excellent for garnishing food). Grapes make pretty vines. Apple pips will grow into little apple trees, and there are all sorts of other things to try, from mangoes to walnuts to avocados. Why not plant a conker or an acorn?

■Become An Organic Gardener

Organic gardening really isn't complicated and peculiar. In fact, it's basically the way people always grew things until the last 40 years or so. Organic gardening means raising your plants without chemical fertilizers, sprays or weedkillers, and fertilizing with natural plant and animal composts.

Chemical fertilizers, herbicides and insecticides have no place in an ecological garden. One benefit is that you no longer have to worry about the poisons in your garden shed. What a relief to know that it is essentially impossible to overdose your plants with liquid seaweed and that you can mix it up in a jug without worrying about residues. (If you have garden chemicals to dispose of, do NOT put them down the drain. Ideally, they would be taken to a special toxic waste collection point, but until one is available you should seal them carefully and put them in your dustbin.)

When most gardening books talk about 'organic' fertilizers what they mean is animal- or plant-based products rather than chemical powders and solutions. Examples are processed manure and garden peat. Most of these will not be organic in the sense of organically raised food. Horse manure from your local stables will contain residues of chemicals from the horses' feed and from worming products. Organic farms depend on good supplies of manure and there is some debate about whether an organic grower should use manure from intensively reared animals, on moral grounds as well as because these manures are likely to be contaminated. Home gardeners can have ready-to-use manure, garden and potting compost from Soil Association standard organic farms delivered anywhere in the UK (see Sources).

SOIL TESTING

Before you start growing edible plants, you may want to have your soil tested. Some town and city soil is badly contaminated with lead from car exhausts, and other heavy metal contamination is possible. Some councils are now regularly testing allotments, and you can send soil samples to Elm Farm Research, a research establishment devoted to organic agriculture. Farmers use their Organic Advisory Service in the process of converting from chemical to organic agriculture.

The home test kits available at nurseries will tell you about pH, nitrogen, phosphate and potash (N-P-K) levels, but organic gardeners recognize that a wide range of trace minerals are important to plants and to human health. This is one reason organically grown food is tastier and more nutritious than food grown with N-P-K chemical fertilizers.

FEEDING THE SOIL

Compost, like 'organic', has more than one meaning. There is the potting mixture which you buy to fill a windowbox. And, vital to the organic gardener, there is compost, which you make yourself from whatever organic materials you have to hand. At home this starts with all your vegetable scraps.

The simplest approach is to mark an area about 4 ft^2, loosen up the soil with a fork and pile on a layer of twigs to keep the bottom aerated, then add whatever you've got whenever it comes along. Sides can be built of scrap timber, if you like, and in wet weather it should be covered with a piece of old carpet. Add grass clippings, leaves, cotton scraps, match sticks, plant clippings, manure, animal litter, anything made of natural materials. (W. G. Shewell Cooper, founder of the Good Gardeners Association, used his old tweed jackets. I have a shabby fox fur coat from a jumble sale which I plan to cut up and put under the straw mulch around my blackcurrants.) Egg shells won't rot, but they are a valuable source of nutrients. Throw them into the compost pile if it suits you or let them dry (on a tray in the oven if you like), crumble them and sprinkle them on the soil, especially on lime-loving plants.

Another possibility is to make a 'green cone' for composting, as shown in the illustration below.

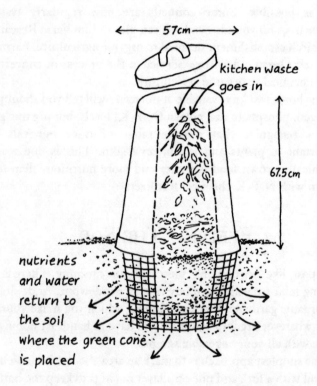

The green cone

Compost needs to be 'activated' with something high in nitrogen. Fresh manure and seaweed work well, comfrey and nettles are both useful, but an even easier and readily available activator is urine. This is perfectly safe, by the way; old timers call it liquid gold.

Leaves are a valuable source of organic matter which is generally wasted. Think of the soft dark leaf mould one finds under trees in a forest. Making your own leaf mould is a better choice than using peat, because it is richer in minerals, available locally and because the 'mining' of bog peat has undesirable ecological consequences. If you can get hold of large quantities of leaves, simply pile them somewhere they can't blow away and leave them until they break down. Or bag the dry leaves in heavy plastic bags and stick them out of the way for a year or two. If you do this each autumn, after the initial wait you will have a steady supply. The annual burning of leaves wastes a wonderful resource.

Seaweed is available in granular or liquid form, and is a potent fertilizer. (Gather your own if you get the chance – put a bucketful of seaweed in the boot when you go to the seaside.) Other useful additions include bracken, wood ashes and paper, hair clippings and spent hops.

A simple way to add nutrients to the soil, smother weeds and cut down on the watering you need to do is to use a mulch. This is a thick layer (you should not be able to see the soil) of some organic material like straw, leafmould or home-made garden compost. A layer of newspaper will help to eradicate perennial weeds.

PEST CONTROL

Keeping insects under control without using dangerous chemicals is not the hurdle you might think. Stronger plants are more disease resistant, and organic gardeners make use of companion planting (tomatoes love carrots) and natural predators like ladybirds. There are a number of sprays and powders available to help you deal with any serious problems. Plain bicarbonate of soda is an effective treatment for mildew (diluted 2 g to 1 litre of water, with a little soft soap to make it stick). A few well-known plant-derived pesticides – derris and pyrethrum – are suitable for organic gardens.

Slugs and snails are probably the worst problem for the organic gardener, and there are many techniques suggested for dealing with them, which range from saucers of beer to night hunts with a torch and a bucketful of soapy water. Place orange or grapefruit shells in the garden. Slugs will gather under them and can be scooped up and disposed of (live burial is effective and drowning is probably most humane). Chemical slug pellets are a well-known danger to birds, which sometimes eat the dead slugs, but this form of pest control has other disadvantages. A study at the Long Ashton Research Station near Bristol suggests that methiocarb, a commonly used slug killer, leads to higher aphid populations because it kills natural aphid predators too.

Weeds are controlled by close planting, mulches and hand weeding. You can use newspapers or old carpets to smother tough perennial weeds and clear ground for planting. Rather than burn the weeds you dig, they can be allowed to dry for a few days (to ensure they don't come to life again) and then added to the compost. Burning is a waste of nutrients and humus, and only necessary for diseased plant material and weed seeds.

Swedish tests have found that stinging nettles make a rich liquid fertilizer which has a better effect on plants than a chemical solution with the same concentration of nutrients. If you have nettles available, simply don gloves and pack them into a bucket or tub, fill with water and cover. Stir every couple of days and after two weeks you can strain off a potent (and smelly) liquid feed for all your plants. Nettle water can be made with fresh or dried nettles, and can be used as a spray to control aphids.

Since Pesticide Regulations 1986 came into force only pesticides on an official list are legal for use, which rules out even tossing your washing-up water over the roses to kill greenfly. Although the Ministry of Agriculture (MAFF) admits that prosecution of home gardeners for using organic pest treatments is unlikely, the situation is nothing short of ridiculous when one considers that in 1986 a senior MAFF official told the House of Commons Agriculture Committee that safety tests on older pesticides may have 'considerable deficiencies in data'. While new tests on these pesticides are being done, a process which could take 20 years, a number of pesticides have been banned after being found to cause birth defects. Until new safety tests are done, suspect chemical pesticides remain legal, while organic plant sprays that have been in use for hundreds of years are technically illegal!

WATER CONSERVATION

Save rainwater and use in the garden or to wash the car – or bicycle. The easiest way is to run water from gutters into a barrel or water butt, which must be carefully covered to ensure that this is not a danger to animals or children. Use plants which don't need to be watered frequently.

Don't water outside during the heat of the day, when the water will evaporate. Occasional deep soakings, rather than frequent sprinkles, save work and water. A mulch (see above, p. 243) will cut watering to a minimum.

PARAPHERNALIA

Try to stick with biodegradable materials when you garden. The average garden centre is full of plastic equipment and tools, plastic pots and polystyrene trays. Grow whatever you can from seed, to avoid buying those plastic pots and get stronger, organically grown seedlings with a far greater choice of variety. Old yoghurt tubs and plastic packing trays are useful for this, and you can cut the bottom off plastic mineral water bottles to make mini-cloches.

Old newspapers can be used to make a home-made version of peat pots. Wrap six or eight sheets around a bottle to form a cylinder and fasten with an 'organic' glue like Gloy. When dry, cut into suitable lengths, place the rings of newspaper in a large garden tray and fill with potting soil. The whole thing can be planted in the garden – roots will grow through the paper.

Choose a biodegradable, untreated gardening string or use strips of cloth to tie up your tomatoes (cloth won't cut into soft stems). Both plants and ties can go straight on to the compost pile.

SEED SAVERS

Current UK legislation (the Plant Seeds and Varieties Act of 1964 and later amending Acts) has virtually eliminated many old varieties by establishing a list of 'approved' seeds. Plant varieties can be patented and royalties collected on seed sales. Unfortunately, the process of getting a seed variety on to a list and keeping it there is expensive, and the registered maintainer of a seed must sell approximately 5000 packets a year to be eligible to stay on the list (5000 packets retailing at 30p apiece would gross £1500: it costs some £800 just to keep the seed on the list).

An estimated 1500 seed varieties had been lost to the British public by 1985 and more are being lost all the time. One firm gives away packets of 'illegal' varieties with orders over a certain value, since selling the seeds would be in breach of the law.

This is a disaster on three counts.

1. Large firms with agrochemical ties are profiting at the expense of smaller, family-run seed companies. In fact, a majority of seed companies are now owned by chemical giants such as ICI.

2. The hybrids sold to commercial growers are the flavourless varieties discussed in Chapter 5, which require large inputs of chemical fertilizers and pesticides. Our environment is polluted, and we get tasteless and less nutritious food into the bargain.

3. Genetic variety is being lost.

Lawrence Hills of the Henry Doubleday Research Association (HDRA) helped Oxfam to found the world's first vegetable gene bank to preserve hundreds of British varieties which have become illegal to sell. He has suggested that a simple legal change would be to exempt all seed varieties older than 50 years from the regulations. Join the HDRA and get more information about the 'Seed Scandal' from them. Then write to your MP. Buy your seeds from the small firms which are campaigning to have this legislation changed.

And save your own seed. Species acclimatize over generations, and by saving your pea and tomato seed you'll eventually have plants that do especially well in your particular region.

How to Save Your Own Seeds

- Start by saving seeds that germinate easily, such as radishes, marigolds and peas. Let a few plants or pods go to seed, and allow the seeds to dry in an airing cupboard or on a sunny kitchen windowsill. Seal them in bags or glass jars.
- Save seed from plants that have done especially well: fruited early, stayed clear of pests and had characteristics you like.
- Scrape out interior seeds like tomato and courgette when completely ripe, remove as much pulp as possible and allow to dry.
- Try old variety seeds available from the HDRA, Suffolk Herbs and other seed preservers, and save your own for future seasons.
- Share with friends, neighbours and seed banks.

Food For The Table

According to John Jeavons, author of *Grow More Vegetables*, it is possible to grow enough vegetables for one person's annual consumption on 100 ft² of ground (that's 10 ft x 10ft, the size of a small bedroom). If you eat a lot of vegetables you might need a bit more room. Double that area and you can also grow a year's supply of soft fruit. And, he says, after the initial hard work, only 5–10 minutes a day will maintain that 100 ft². Sounds enticing? Novice gardeners, on neglected city soil, can't expect those yields, but Jeavons recommends that you start with 100 ft² anyway. Many domestic gardens have a plot this big which could be devoted to vegetable growing.

As an urban farmer, I've always concentrated on speciality crops – the things which I can't find at the shop or which are very expensive – and I buy bulky crops like potatoes, carrots and onions from an organic farm.

When you put in trees and shrubs, consider varieties that offer crops as a bonus. Fruit trees, grape vines and quince bushes (which have lovely pink and white flowers, and sulphur-coloured fruit which is excellent in pies and jam) are favourites. Or let the brambles grow at the bottom of the garden and give them a little manure in the spring (you might prefer to plant cultivated blackberry varieties to get a higher yield).

Tuck herbs in among your flowers, in beds and in windowboxes. Try to keep some parsley, mint and other favourite herbs near the kitchen; you won't use them half as often if you have to trek to the other end of the back garden. Food plants can be grown in hanging baskets, windowboxes and tubs, indoors and out.

ALLOTMENTS

A growing number of young people, women and people from a wide variety of backgrounds – managers as well as the urban unemployed – are now taking on allotments. There has been a resurgence of interest in this form of agriculture, which dates back to Elizabethan times and was particularly associated with 'digging for victory' during the Second World War. People turn to allotments for exercise, fresh air and fresh food, and for a sense of connection with the land. An allotment gives everyone a chance to have abundant organic vegetables at minimal cost.

If you have never seen anyone gardening and never done any

yourself, be cautious about taking on an allotment by yourself. For the first year or two it will be rather like a baby, needing lots of attention and feeding. Old timers may be helpful but they sometimes resent newcomers and new-fangled techniques like mulching.

There are lots of people who like the idea of growing their own, but they often fail because they take on too much, too soon, and they don't put enough time into acquiring basic information and skills.

Keep the following points in mind.

1. The closer your allotment is to your home, the more often you will visit it.

2. If you haven't gardened much before, try to start with a small plot, no more than 10 ft² if possible.

3. Share a plot or pair of plots with a friend. You can cover each other over holidays and provide moral support during bad weather.

4. Don't overspend; new gardeners tend to go a little mad buying equipment and seeds.

5. Find out who organizes and administers the allotments. Try to meet the other allotment holders, who can tell you about the soil, sources of manure and so on.

6. Look at what is growing well in other plots for clues as to promising crops, but don't stick to cabbages and potatoes just because everyone else does. Most allotments will not be organically run but many gardeners are receptive to organic methods.

FLOWERS

Faced with a bare garden, the first thing one does is head for the garden centre to buy trays of pansies and wallflowers. Then you pull them out and plant something else the next season. This is what I call the municipal gardens approach, which is wasteful and a lot of work compared to a closely planted perennial bed.

Plant old-fashioned scented varieties, which are enjoying something of a revival thanks to interest in the traditional English garden. Modern hybrid roses appeal to some, but the glorious fragrances of 'old' roses will be a delight to everyone who comes into your garden and you'll be helping to preserve genetic diversity. Like vegetables, flowers have been bred for size and appearance in recent years, and more subtle charms have been neglected. But even the big seed companies offer a few of the old-fashioned varieties and there are specialist firms with fabulous ranges.

If you have room, grow plenty of flowers for cutting. Even a small garden can offer quite a good supply of house flowers, especially if you use plenty of greenery too – much nicer than those plastic-wrapped bundles of imported flowers most of us depend on to add some colour to the table, and organically grown too, unlike the flowers we buy (an estimated 20 per cent of the pesticides used on Colombian flowers, a major source for UK florists, are banned in Europe).

The floral industry uses more pesticides than any other agricultural business because, they say, consumers are even more reluctant to accept flowers which are less than perfect than they are apples or cabbages. Florists use vast quantities of plastic containers and accessories, synthetic fabric flowers and ribbons, balloons, paints and dyes, as well as floral preservatives. Cost margins are slim, as traditional floral shops compete with mass-market supermarket floral departments, and most commercial flowers are imported out of season flowers, or exotics. Encourage your florist to use locally grown flowers, simply constructed arrangements and ask about the pesticides used on the flowers you buy.

A well-designed picking garden can give you flowers throughout most of the year. When you grow your own flowers, plant sturdy native species and harvest in the evening directly into a bucket of clean water. Allow the flowers to sit overnight in a cool, dark place before arranging them.

TREES

The loss of forests, both temperate and tropical, is one of the twentieth century's greatest disasters. Trees have a special place in human consciousness – in Jungian psychology they stand for wholeness. Most of us can remember a tree or two, perhaps from childhood, which played a special part in our lives. For me, there is the apple tree at my grandpa's where I could hide with a book and eat green fruit all afternoon.

In nature, trees grow where soil, light, wind and moisture suit them, but in towns they have to struggle to grow where they are planted. (As we found in the storm of 1987, many trees were vulnerable because they lacked a balancing, buttressing spread of roots.)

Architect Christopher Alexander suggests that urban trees need people as much as people need trees. They should be planted where they provide not just attractive greenery but shade during hot spells, a pleasant spot for a seat or a good place for children to play, because this means that the people who enjoy them will also care for them. Plant a tree whenever you can.

THE ORGANIC LAWN

Lawns are something of a dilemma for an organic gardener. An immaculate turf requires either enormous labour or heavy application of herbicides – some people turn into fiendish chemists at the sight of a cheerful little creeping buttercup. And environmentalists concerned about famine say that we should devote the land given over to purely ornamental lawns to growing food. There are lots of attractive ways to incorporate food growing into even a front garden (what about a thickly planted bed of potatoes, with their lush foliage and pretty flowers?).

LAWN TIPS

- Choose an appropriate seed blend. A hard-wearing mixture will be easier to maintain (and the weeds won't be quite so obvious).
- Minimize the lawn area. All most of us want is a pleasant stretch of green for sunbathing and the smaller the area you have to maintain the easier it will be to use organic methods.
- Allow extra lawn space to go wild, or plant an easy to maintain wildflower lawn, or plant another groundcover.
- Set your (non-electric) mower blades to 2 in. Lawns do best if cut fairly high, but frequently.
- Leave lawn clippings where they fall, to replenish the soil. (Unless there are too many, in which case they will stick to your feet and get tracked into the house.)
- Remember that worms are good for the soil. Sweep the castings around on a dry day. Spike the lawn – with a fork or with spiked boots available from gardening shops.
- Feed it with a high-nitrogen natural fertilizer two or three times a year. Seaweed meal is very good and so is sifted compost.
- Arm yourself with an old kitchen knife to dig out dandelions and dock. Or you can leave the dandelions, eat the early sprouts in salad and make the flowers into wine.

PAVING

If you decide to increase your amount of paved area, don't concrete it. Approximately one-third of the land in an average city is already concrete or asphalt, mostly for roads and car parks, and this has undesirable ecological consequences. Solid paving leads to water run-off because natural drainage is blocked, affects the microclimate and does nothing useful with the solar energy which falls on it. Damage can only be repaired by replacing the whole slab (instead of just a couple of bricks) and it essentially kills the soil below.

Make a surface with old bricks or paving stones, set in dirt so that mosses and plants can grow between the cracks. This sort of surface responds well to weathering – it will look better in ten years than it does now. The delicate ecology of earthworms, plant and insect life will be preserved, while you still have a firm, dry surface on which to put a table or for children to push a tricycle. Paths can be laid in the same way, or you can use stepping stones set in grass or low-growing plants.

Traditional York stone (often advertised in the Classified section of the newspaper) is laid on a foundation of crushed stone, rolled flat, which allows water to drain away without turning the soil into mud, a good idea with any material on a damp site. Rather than point the cracks, place the stones quite closely together and allow tiny plants to grow. Stonemasons think well-laid unequally sized rectangles of York stone makes the best paved surface, but consider old London paving a good second best and, for something cheaper, reconstituted Cotswold stone slabs. But cement-based paving is not as durable as stone, which will last virtually for ever. Old bricks are attractive, but you must ensure that they are of outdoor quality (or frost will crack them).

OUTDOOR LIVING

If you want to use your garden all year round, it needs to be congenial. Children need toys that can be brought out quickly when there is a clear afternoon, and some flowers or green things will make you feel brighter too – and provide something to cut and bring inside. Provide as much natural seating as you can, which can stay in place all year round. The lawn is fine on warm, dry summer days, but you'll use the garden a lot more if there are sheltered, sunny seats for cool weather. A bench is lovely, if your garden is big enough. Thick sawn logs are good too. Think about shelter from the sun and about whether you want the seat to face activity or to be more secluded. Shelter from wind is important much of the year and a big umbrella will help during hot weather. Make the garden an outdoor room, connected to the house, with a table, chairs, play equipment and shelves. An accessible storage place is vital if you have wood and canvas folding chairs, and for toys.

Privacy has a great deal to do with how much we use our gardens. It is not rude to want privacy from even the friendliest of neighbours, but some diplomacy is a good idea. An 8-ft board fence is not diplomatic. And whatever you plant, think about how it will affect your neighbours – don't cut off their light. Climbing plants are very useful, on a trellis or on wires.

White flowers show up at dusk and after dark, so if you are going to use your garden then it is well worth concentrating on white blooms. Some form of lighting will make the garden more enticing on mild evenings.

A free-standing greenhouse is an efficient way of using solar energy, but if it is connected to the house you have an extra room, as well as a place to grow seedlings and houseplants (which you can tend in the winter without going outdoors). A conservatory is a sort of greenhouse, and most usefully brings the outside and inside together.

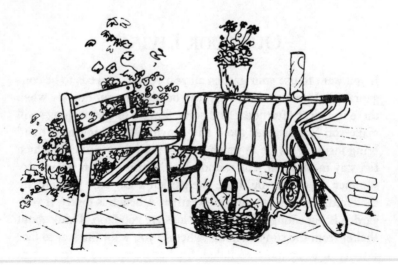

GROWING CHILDREN

Gardening books always warn you that you'll have to choose between your flowers and your children. But why not design the garden to cope with children? Establish a part where no trespassing is allowed for your more tender plants, put a simple fence around the vegetable patch, and watch out for prickly plants and dangerous ones if you have babies around. (I don't see why one couldn't use prickly plants as a harmless deterrent to rough ten year olds.)

Then plant a tough lawn, put up whatever equipment seems appropriate, a sandpit, a low table for children (those big wooden cable reels can do for this – and they're great to roll around). Hang a tyre swing or just a rope to climb.

Children love to dig and plant. You can hardly get them started too early, with plenty of help and encouragement, and their own collection of pots or a designated area for their own garden.

The easiest way to protect precious flower beds is to raise them, although it will require some initial hard work and a lot of extra soil. Use stone or brick to make a rough seat at the front and you'll find tending the beds a lot easier on your back. The flowers are close so you can smell them easily and children can look at them without scrabbling through your nicest hostas.

Organize a shared back garden, especially nice if you live in a place where each garden is only a narrow sliver. This could be an open area between six or eight houses, with a play area for the kids.

WILDLIFE GARDENING

Domestic gardens can provide extra habitat for beleaguered creatures whose natural habitats are being chewed up by development. And because a certain amount of casualness is necessary to make the right environment, this type of garden should appeal to occasional gardeners. That bed of nettles is there for the butterflies, of course, not because you never have gloves on when you go into the garden.

There are a number of books available on this subject (see Sources) and local wildlife trusts can advise on suitable plants for your area, but here are a few ideas.

1. Set up a bird table or hang a feeder. Put it somewhere you can see it from the house, but out of reach of cats. The Royal Society for the Protection of Birds (RSPB) has a number of helpful factsheets and leaflets.

2. Plant native trees and shrubs, which support a wide range of insect life. This in turn attracts birds, hedgehogs, frogs and toads – an ecological cycle in the making! Hedges provide a home for many creatures. Prune trees like hawthorn into an excellent thick hedge. Try to place these as a windbreak, which will perhaps cut your heating bills as well as make sheltered spots in the garden. (The RSPB has an information sheet on trees and shrubs for birds.)

3. Plant native wildflowers – these include snowdrops, blue-bells, violets and primroses, as well as poppies, cornflowers and ox-eye daisies.

4. A wildflower lawn, like many native plants, grows best on poor soil. You'll need to clear perennial weeds before you start and continue to weed until the native plants are established. This sort of lawn needs mowing only twice a year!

5. Plant to attract bees and butterflies and birds. They like old-fashioned, sweet-scented cottage flowers. Buddleia, which grows wild on decaying inner city roofs, is known as the 'butterfly bush'. Birds like berries and, part of your organic gardening programme, insects.

Piles of rocks, bricks or logs will make a home for many small creatures like beetles and centipedes, and maybe even a hedge-hog. Think what a wonderful garden you'll have for scientifically-minded children.

Leave the weeds. This is so tempting that it could easily get out of hand, but try setting aside one area for nettles and buttercups (or whatever grows where you are). My garden is too small to allow much of this, but I can't resist my patch of creeping buttercup. I know they're invasive, but they look so beautiful in a dark corner that I only sporadically try to uproot them. Minimize tidying up. Don't clear away piles of brush, spent growth, fallen leaves. A healthy ecosystem needs all stages of growth and decay.

Build a pond. The easiest way to line it is with a rubber liner. You can put in a variety of water plants and either wait for the insects to come, or get a bucketful of water and mud from a friend's pond to start yours off with water boatmen, water beetles and snails. Apparently frogs will find their own way, but if you are in a hurry you can import some from your friend (not from the wild). Frogs and toads include slugs in their diet, another ecological boon. Their habitat is declining in the countryside, so friendly gardens are important for their survival. (Obviously you need to take special precautions with a pond if you have children.)

CULTIVATING A GREEN THUMB

▶ Garden with someone else if you possibly can. It doesn't matter if they know as little as you to start with. The important thing is to have someone to show the emergent sweet peas, to commiserate over aphid damage and to share the initial spadework.

▶ Take it easy. Don't put your back out with improvident digging (make sure tool handles are long enough, bend your knees and not your back, turn to throw the spadeful of soil after you have straightened up – and don't try to do the whole patch in one afternoon).

▶ Wearing gloves helps to prevent blisters. Sticking your fingers in handcream, Vaseline or butter will make cleaning much easier (make sure the cream goes under your fingernails), and a hat and/or sunscreen will protect your neck and nose.

▶ Buy or borrow decent tools and learn to care for them. Wellies aren't exactly tools but they come first (or sturdy country shoes which can take a battering and which you won't worry about). A good fork won't get bent first time out and an expensive pair of clippers will last for ever. Start with a fairly narrow spade or a fork if your soil is really heavy (you'll want to have both eventually), a small trowel, a hoe, a pair of clippers, a mower if you have a lawn (power mowers are unnecessary for modest domestic lawns).

▶ Get advice. Watch TV programmes about gardening and join the HDRA. You may also want to become a member of the Royal Horticultural Society for their monthly magazine, free advice and entry to shows.

▶ Read, especially during the winter. Organic gardening is a popular topic, and books in print range from profusely illustrated coffee table books to small manuals on specific techniques. Many gardening writers tend towards an organic approach nowadays, and some newspaper gardening columns are excellent and of course usefully seasonal. They often list gardens open to the public.

▶ Look at other people's gardens. Every neighbourhood has a few keen gardeners, and they are often delighted to know that you admire the fruits of their labours and ready to give tips on dealing with your area's quirks of sun or soil.

▶ There is also a National Gardens Scheme, in which people with particularly fine gardens open them to the public on a day or two (many are open more often than that). National Trust gardens will prove inspiring. At Sissinghurst each plant is labelled so you can write down the names of the plants you like.

▶ Visit organic gardens. The HDRA runs Ryton Gardens, a demonstration organic garden on 22 acres near Coventry, and there is a demonstration organic garden at the Centre for Alternative Technology in Wales.

▶ Grow your own plants from seed. This saves money, gives you a wider choice and stronger organically grown plants.

▶ Learn to propagate from cuttings and how to layer plants. An experienced gardening friend is a great help.

▶ Plant plenty of bulbs (deeper than you think, and put a handful of bonemeal in the bottom of each hole). They get each new season off to a good start.

GARDENING SIMPLIFIED

- Dig your garden near the house.
- Tackle a small area at a time.
- Use easy techniques.
- Live and let live: don't worry about a little insect damage unless you're showing at the Chelsea Flower Show.
- Grow things you love to eat or smell.
- Mix flowers and vegetables, and herbs and fruit in the same bed.

HANDS TO EARTH

Environmentalists often seem to view the world in an abstract way, quite different from the focused attention of the amateur naturalist who loves nature in the particular – the twist of a tree root over a rock outcropping, the hum of beetles in a particular grove on a summer's night. For this reason, tending a garden is an important part of home ecology. Growing green things gives us a chance to make a tangible, living difference in the world around us. We join the community of gardeners, who have around the world and through the centuries tended the earth, produced food and created beauty.

Think of it: working in the garden is the only time most of us ever put our hand to the earth, touching the surface of our planet. The environment ceases to be an abstraction when you feel soil crumble between your fingers, watch the winds and weather and light, and pay attention to the tiny miracles of the natural world outside your door.

16

Nurturing Our Children

Pregnancy brings many physical changes, but perhaps even more dramatic are the changes in one's plans and priorities. Yet parenthood often jogs us into a new awareness of the world and a new concern about the environment we live in. This was true for me. I began to pay attention to news stories about air pollution and magazine articles about pesticides in food when I was pregnant with my first child. I wanted to be as healthy as possible for my child, and the future seemed more tangible, more relevant, with new life growing inside me. Indeed, there are many ecological aspects to childbearing and childrearing; as time passes, as my children grow older, I have begun to learn new lessons as I answer their questions about the world around.

Choosing To Have Children

Population has always been an important issue for environmentalists. Human beings put great pressure on the earth and restricting our numbers is a vital part of improving our prospects. The 1994 Cairo Population Summit provoked much debate about family planning in third world countries. There are those who advocate improved access to contraception as the primary tool for reducing population and those who emphasize poverty reduction, improvements in the status of women, or economic development.

This polarization may obscure the fact that women around the world want to be able to choose whether or not to have children, and improved birth control options are important to all of us. No option is perfect. Hormonal methods like the pill and other forms of contraception are associated with a range of health problems (as is repeated pregnancy). Abortion is an essential part of an effective reproductive health care system, but it should be the option of last resort. Voluntary sterilization is effective and relatively cheap, but it is not reversible and has not always been voluntary.

Foresight, the pre-conceptual care organization, recommends natural family planning (NFP) as the healthiest method of contraception because it uses no artificial aids at all (see Sources). To follow NFP, a woman charts her ovulation cycle by keeping a record of her temperature, cervical shape and vaginal mucus. These change very regularly throughout the menstrual cycle and most women find that they can recognise their own patterns with great accuracy after several months' practice. The method requires diligence and motivation; its success rate is roughly comparable to using a diaphragm with spermicide.

Otherwise, condoms are probably the healthiest, most environmentally sound method as long as they are properly disposed of in rubbish meant for landfill, not flushed down the lavatory where they can end up choking birds and fish.

PRE-CONCEPTION CARE

Foresight has been at the forefront of pre-conceptual care, giving advice and information about the environmental factors affecting foetal health with the aim of reducing the problems of birth defects and infant ill-health. It provides material on nutrition, pollution, allergies and natural family planning, and can refer you to a doctor who runs a Foresight clinic if you would like a full health check – including hair analysis for heavy metal contamination – before you conceive.

If you are already pregnant Foresight can give advice on diet, nutritional supplements, protecting yourself and your baby from pollution, and combating allergies. Foresight also advises couples who are having difficulty in conceiving, and publishes an excellent little booklet on additives which you can tuck into your wallet, each E number colour-coded for quick reference.

PREPARING FOR BIRTH

The overwhelming feeling of responsibility for another life leaves a first-time mother vulnerable to pressure, especially from those who are providing antenatal care. The following information and contacts should help you to resolve questions for yourself.

Your doctor or midwife, as well as any good book on pregnancy will recommend a healthy diet with plenty of fresh fruit and vegetables, and will caution against tobacco, alcohol and drugs. But you are unlikely to be warned that pregnant women should also avoid hazardous household chemicals. Your nose will tip you off about some of these – many pregnant women find that their sense of smell becomes particularly acute. Pesticides, chemical fertilizers, many cleaning products, paints and paint thinners, contact adhesive and all aerosols are best removed from your home – Chapter 12 suggests alternatives for many standard products. Even hair dyes have been shown to be carcinogenic and mutagenic in laboratory tests. Small amounts are absorbed through the scalp and the fumes are inhaled. For several years US obstetricians have been warning pregnant women against using any chemical hair treatment.

These changes are also important after your baby is born, because of ingestion through your breastmilk and directly. Many babies grow up surrounded by dangerous fumes from household disinfectants, used out of misplaced concern about hygiene. Most disinfectants contain chemicals which can affect the central nervous system and cause organ damage.

Avoid all medication (many common drugs have been shown to have a deleterious effect on the developing foetus), and make a special effort to stay away from food additives, including artificial sweeteners. Organic fruits and vegetables are not contaminated with pesticide residues so buy them if you can, and if you eat meat, try to get organically grown meat, or choose only lean cuts. Pesticides, hormones and antibiotics concentrate in fatty tissue. Tea and coffee, as well as alcohol, should be treated with caution while you're expecting, and while you are planning to conceive.

PRENATAL TESTING

The use of high frequency sound waves to monitor pregnancy has become routine in Britain, in spite of the fact that there have been no long-term studies done to establish its safety. Critics of universal scanning say that no form of technological intervention should be used as a matter of routine and that dependence on information from scans means that practitioners have less incentive really to listen to women. In addition midwives and doctors are losing their palpation skills because of over-reliance on machine data. Correct reading of ultrasound is difficult. Even in a controlled study done by the Royal College of Obstetricians and Gynaecologists one normal foetus was aborted after an incorrect diagnosis.

No one knows what effect scanning has on an unborn baby, but unusual foetal activity is common afterwards. Research continues to find that babies in the womb are more sensitive than previously supposed, with senior researchers now advising an anaesthetic for foetuses before mothers are given amniocentesis tests.

Routine scanning is expensive, upwards of £20 million a year in Britain, not including the cost of equipment. No research data is kept on women and babies exposed to scanning, and the World Health Organization has issued a policy statement stressing that 'ultrasound screening during pregnancy is now in widespread use without sufficient evaluation'.

Even amniocentesis and chorionic villus sampling (CVS), aimed at catching congenital defects in time to allow for an abortion, give uncertain results and sometimes cause problems where there were none. Sometimes testing is justified simply on the grounds that it reassures parents, who have become increasingly jumpy about the process of pregnancy and childbirth.

A Natural Birth

The way we give birth is an ecological issue because proponents of modern birth technologies tend to see the ability to bear children, one of the primary cycles of the natural world, as insufficient and inefficient. The explosion of interest in natural childbirth in the last two decades is a sign that women are unwilling to see birth as simply an arduous medical procedure.

One of the ways the medical profession took control of maternal services was to make birth, which had always taken place at home and within the community, a hospital procedure.

In fact, a recent study at the Institute of Epidemiology and Health Services at Leeds University found that the presence of a supportive spouse or midwife during labour does more to reduce the need for caesarean and forceps deliveries than does technological 'active management'. Perhaps the most important factor in a successful labour is that the woman in labour feels comfortable and confident about her own abilities, and at ease in her surroundings. It's no coincidence that some women arrive at hospital only to have their contractions stop. This is embarrassing and inconvenient, but hardly surprising. If you were to move a labouring animal, the same natural safety mechanism would come into effect.

You are far more likely to end up with what is euphemistically called a 'managed labour' – with electronic foetal monitoring, artificial breaking of waters and the use of hormones to speed labour – in hospital. There are a number of reasons for this. A woman who isn't at ease is more likely to need intervention, hospital routine makes a timetable for labour more likely, and the simple fact that equipment, drugs and staff are available makes it more likely that they will be used. There is also an apt expression, the 'cascade of management', used to describe the way one act of intervention leads to another. If your waters are manually ruptured to speed up labour, the contractions become much more painful and you are therefore more likely to need or want drugs or an epidural. If labour is induced, you cannot move around freely, and will probably have a more difficult and painful time, making the use of further drugs more likely. If a woman has anaesthetics, she is more likely to need a forceps delivery and so on.

Many couples think that they aren't allowed to have their baby at home, but in fact community midwives are obliged by law to attend any birth in their area, and there are a number of organizations which will help you if you want to have a home birth (see Sources).

BREASTFEEDING

Only 64 per cent of British mothers choose to breastfeed their babies at all and of that number only 40 per cent (26 per cent of the total) continue to breastfeed for at least four months, the minimum period recommended by most paediatricians. A recent survey showed a slight decline in the number of breastfeeding mothers over the past decade.

Breastfeeding is officially encouraged through the government's Breast is Best campaign, but not nearly enough is done to make it easy for many new mothers. Midwives and nurses try to help, but hospital routine doesn't make early breastfeeding easy and the standard advice is that 'It'll be better when you get home'.

Many of us give up nursing because we haven't got enough milk. Why is this? The main problem is extremely simple: not allowing the baby to nurse enough. The sucking is what stimulates milk production. You also need to eat well and get enough rest. Midwives and doctors will give you advice on feeding your baby, but they still tell mothers how many minutes to nurse on each breast and how often to feed – rules which have nothing to do with what your baby needs.

Taking the baby to bed with you can make things much easier – ask your midwife, or your health visitor, about this after the birth. Young children, and older children and adults too, often feel isolated if they sleep alone, but many parents feel a misplaced sense of guilt about the fact that their children like to climb into bed with them. A large 'family' bed is a happy option for some, and a low bed (or futon) is a great help, especially with a small baby. See Sources for more information.

The other factor which prevents women breastfeeding is embarrassment about using their breasts in this way and particularly about the difficulty of feeding in public. Social support, from partners, family and friends, is terribly important in successful breastfeeding. Women who will happily bare their breasts on a beach are sometimes desperately shy about feeding a baby, no matter how discreetly. Perhaps this is because they feel that they are the only one! We so rarely see a mother breastfeeding that it doesn't seem normal or ordinary and any use of our breasts is treated as something sexual. The more common breastfeeding becomes, and the more comfortable all of us (men, women and children) become about it, the easier it will be for every new mother. (The fact that women who breastfeed are less likely to suffer from breast cancer should be an additional inducement.)

NAPPIES

When you have a leaky baby you get obsessed with nappies. Fathers swop notes on the best type, and friends report on which shop has your favourite brand at 50p off. Of course I'm talking about disposable plastic-and-paper nappies, not the terry nappies our mothers or grandmothers boiled in a copper. Sixty-five per cent of babies are put into disposable nappies and approximately nine million are used every day in Britain – used and discarded. But disposable nappies simply are not disposable. They are non-degradable, a potential health hazard, and they contribute to the depletion of limited timber and petroleum reserves. It is estimated that 4 per cent of household solid waste is made up of soiled nappies. For every pound we spend on disposable nappies, tax-payers will spend 10p on disposal.

I understand why people use disposables, and I have used them myself. After all, everyone else seems to, including the maternity ward at your local hospital. This tacit medical endorsement, fortified by the free samples given to new mothers, is enough to convince many parents. Because disposables save time and effort they can seem worth the expense, though it is considerable: some £1500 for a child potty-trained by the age of two-and-a-half.

Modern sanitation involves the separation of sewage from other waste, but with disposable nappies huge amounts of faecal matter are treated as part of the household rubbish rather than being processed through the sewage system. Indeed, nappies may be yet another source of groundwater contamination from land-fill sites. 'Leachate containing viruses from human faeces (including live vaccines from routine childhood immunizations) can leak into the earth and pollute underground water supplies', concluded a study by disposal specialist Carl Lehrburger.

Nappy rash was virtually unknown before plastic pants became common in the 1950s, and the mother whose child has a recurrently raw and painful bottom will know that it is essential to get the child out of 'ordinary', i.e. disposable, nappies. Doctors suggest leaving the child bare as much as possible (a good rule for any baby) and at least temporarily switching to cloth nappies.

■Cloth Tips

Terry nappies are very absorbent, but the standard 24 in squares can be awkward to handle and pin. The new fitted cloth nappies, with shaped nylon covers, are easier to use. Although the initial expense of using cloth nappies and covers is much greater than buying a bag of disposables at the supermarket, in the long run you should cut costs by about half, even taking laundering into account, and subsequent babies add nothing to the total.

With modern washing machines and dryers, using cloth nappies should be much easier for us than it was for past generations. Here's how.

1. Make sure you have enough nappies, 3 to 4 dozen. You will also need a covered pail to hold rinsed nappies, a supply of borax and a gentle washing powder. Gauze liners make cleaning easier – use them rather than disposable paper liners.

2. Half fill the pail with a mild borax solution to disinfect the nappies, and reduce odours and staining.

3. Wet nappies can go straight into the nappy pail – or rinse them first – and soiled nappies should be shaken or scraped (with an old knife or spoon) and then rinsed in the lavatory bowl first.

4. Before putting in the washing machine, drain the excess solution into the lavatory, then use a spin cycle to drain dirty water. Then use a hot wash, and double rinse – don't overload the machine.

5. Tumble drying on high heat will help sterilization and makes the nappies softer than drying on a rack or over a radiator. Dry outside whenever you can: sunlight acts as a natural disinfectant and gentle bleach.

6. Try to avoid plastic pants. Terry nappies can sometimes be used on their own. 'Soakers' are knitted wool or fabric covers which offer moderate protection.

7. Let your baby go bare whenever you can, both inside and out.

8. Don't feel guilty about using a disposable occasionally. But avoid those scented plastic bags made to wrap disposables for disposal!

The Women's Environmental Network, or the *Yellow Pages*, can help you find a nappy service. The cost falls between washing your own and using disposables. A nappy service provides cloth nappies, and regular pick-up and collection. You hand over your pail of rinsed nappies, and in return get a pile of fresh ones, washed and dried in high-temperature machines.

THE BABY MARKET

It is easy to get carried away dressing a small child. The miniature trappings are very appealing, but they cost a small fortune and have to be replaced every couple of months as a baby grows. Chapter 3 has general ideas about ecological buying and the suggestions about buying second-hand become especially relevant. You may be lucky enough to be given a nearly-new baby wardrobe (and it's well worth letting people know that you are not averse to borrowing clothes and baby gear). Otherwise, charity shops and boot sales sometimes throw up terrific bargains. Tiny clothes get very little wear so they are often in excellent condition. You may well find you can afford far better quality – and originally more expensive – clothes by careful shopping. You'll be staggered at the amount of money you can save by buying second-hand. Encourage friends and relatives to ask before they buy presents, so they can supplement your 'finds' instead of duplicating them.

When your child has outgrown his or her clothes, and you are not saving them for another baby, either pass them on to someone or donate them to one of the charity shops.

Baby equipment, too, can be acquired second-hand. Check your National Childbirth Trust (NCT) branch newsletter, local newspaper and the notices in the newsagent's window, or place your own advertisement. Be prepared to give your purchases a good scrub and check first for the small parts which may be missing or broken, and practically impossible to replace.

SAFETY

Although we worry about children getting hold of drain cleaner or methylated spirits, the most common type of 'poison' is medication. Many drugs, both prescription and over-the-counter, look very much like sweets, and this is another excellent reason for cutting down on the drugs you use.

▶ Read labels and take their warnings seriously.

▶ Keep dangerous items well out of reach – not on the bathroom shelf or in your handbag.

▶ Because of its high alcohol content, a few spoonfuls of your cologne could lead to unconsciousness and even death for a small child.

▶ Get rid of whatever you can – aerosol cans of fly killer, old medicines and unwanted aftershave.

▶ Return unused drugs to the chemist for disposal.

▶ Switch to safe household products and toiletries. Even with these, care is advisable.

▶ DIY items are probably the most hazardous things you'll have around the house. Lock them away.

IMMUNIZATION

Most health care professionals insist that universal immunization is both safe and necessary. They tell parents, for example, that there's a clear choice between having measles and having a vaccine. However, a 1978 survey found that more than half the children who contracted measles had been vaccinated against it, and a study at the Primal Health Research Centre in the UK, led by Michel Odent, found that there was five times the incidence of asthma, a modern plague among schoolchildren, in those who had received the whooping cough vaccine. Vaccines are intended to work on the body's immunological system and it is not surprising there could be side-effects like this.

While reassuring the public that all is well with current immunization programmes, the medical profession and governments are looking for alternatives, obviously aware that present risks are not entirely acceptable.

A common justification for universal vaccination is that it is largely responsible for this century's reduction in infant mortality. The common childhood diseases were, however, in decline before many modern vaccines came on the scene. Better hygiene, clean water and an improved diet were crucial factors.

If you have a young baby, take the time to look into this question before you make up your mind. Your clinic (or GP or health visitor) will press you to have the baby's first set of shots at two months, but the timing is not crucial – they like to start at this age because you are still bringing the child into the clinic regularly.

The possible risks with the whooping cough vaccine have received a great deal of attention, but there are concerns about other routine vaccinations. One might think that a sickly infant would need immunization more than a robust child, but children who are already unwell are most vulnerable to ill-effects from vaccination. An American study shows a connection between the DPT vaccine and cot-death – the most likely explanation being that in these cases the vaccine was the last straw for a child whose system was already under stress.

An Australian doctor has used vitamin C and zinc supplements to boost immune function before giving vaccines to vulnerable Aboriginal children, and infant mortality in that group virtually disappeared. If you decide to go ahead with vaccination, you might want to give your baby extra vitamin C and some multi-mineral drops containing zinc.

A CHILD'S DIET

Many parents seem to think, perhaps thanks to the baby food industry, that children need and like to eat a limited range of 'children's food'. They give the children an early tea of fish fingers and mashed potatoes, and later eat something far more interesting themselves. Is it such a surprise that children become 'fussy' and refuse to try anything different.

A child's palate is more sensitive than ours, but it is easy to get into the habit of adding strong spices to food after setting aside a portion for the little ones (this takes a little juggling with some recipes). Letting children eat with you (from the age of six months they can begin to join in family meals) is quite an incentive to improve your own eating habits!

Recent analyses of schoolchildren's diets have shown startling cases of malnourishment. British children not only eat far too much sugar and fat but are short of major quantifiable nutrients. They are spending more than £220 million a year on sweets and snacks on their way to and from secondary schools, and are developing eating habits based on grazing, quick fix snacks with little nutritive content.

There's no doubt that changing your child's diet is even harder than changing your own. Move cautiously and make sure that you are willing to stop eating crisps, or whatever it might be, too. There are bound to be some 'good' foods your children like. Carrot sticks? Apple sauce? Cheese? How about vegetables? Try cutting up salad ingredients very finely and use a creamy (perhaps yoghurt-based) dressing. Or cut up raw vegetables (celery, red and green peppers, carrots, fennel, cauliflower, tomatoes, young turnips) into pieces for nibbling – it's a good idea to keep a plentiful supply of these crudités in the fridge. They are good for adults too. Serve with a dip occasionally.

The sugar industry is immensely powerful, as Professor John Yudkin graphically details in a new edition of the classic *Pure, White and Deadly*. Sugar has been implicated in some cancers, liver disease, gout and eye and skin problems, as well as in diabetes. Yudkin asserts that 'If only a small fraction of what is known about sugar was revealed in connection with any other material used as a food additive, that material would be banned.'

Sucrose is not the only form of sugar. Quite a few manufacturers are now substituting other sweeteners to mislead parents trying to avoid refined sugar. Fruit syrups can also rot teeth, but they are not so concentrated as refined white sugar and provide some nutrients along with sweetening power. Dove Farm sells a range of sugar-free biscuits made with organic flour that offer a persuasive substitute for the supermarket version.

Here are some general guidelines for eating with children.

1.   Let your child join in with your meals from about the age of six months, with tiny tastes of suitable foods.

2. Eat a variety of foods, both cooked and raw.

3. Don't force anything on a child.

4. Aim for a balanced diet over the course of each week, not each day.

5. Don't panic if your child doesn't eat as much as you think he or she should; a healthy child will not starve him or herself!

6. Don't let a child who isn't eating meals have sweets and crisps.

7. Notice which nutritious foods your child likes, and try to emphasize those dishes.

8. Let children get involved in planning and preparation as early as possible.

Many older children will be fascinated by food and development issues – you can talk about additives and pesticides, visit city farms and discuss where our food comes from, and how what we eat affects people in other countries.

Growing at least a little of your food is another way to get children involved in family meals. Do everything you can to encourage cooking skills (even when this means helping to deal with flour on the ceiling afterwards). One of the most interesting things you can do is make or bake common shop-bought foods: water biscuits, for example, or digestives or baked beans.

Play And Playthings

Babies have cupboards full of battery-driven stuffed dogs and helicopters with revolving blades. Even good old Lego comes with ready-made detail nowadays. These toys are designed for what one box describes as 'imaginative play' – that is, play the way the designer imagines it, not play which genuinely encourages a child's imagination.

What effect does this have on children? Some will grow up wanting an endless supply of new toys. Others will annoy their parents by ignoring their toys and pulling out all the saucepans for a jam session in the corner. Parents are apt to lose their temper when an expensive toy is taken apart 'to find out how it works'. But if you give a small child a toy with complicated internal mechanisms, native curiosity (the imagination we want to encourage) inspires the child to set to work with a screwdriver.

Older children compare notes with friends at school, and the child with the wrong bicycle or wrong computer software feels left out and out of step. How a child copes with this depends on their own independence and self-confidence, and on whether their parents also feel the need to have every new gadget.

The environmental and social consequences of this are profound. The sheer quantity of raw materials used to make toys (most of which don't last for long) is one aspect of the problem. Even more important are the lessons children learn before they can walk about ceaseless consumption, ready-made entertainment and disposability.

The ability to develop close relationships in later life is closely linked to childhood friendships. Some studies suggest that other children are even more important than the mother in a child's emotional development. Children need to spend informal time together, not only school time or organized visits. This can be difficult, depending on where you live and whether there are other children of roughly the same age nearby. There are no easy solutions, but it may be that an overdependence on toys has a lot to do with not having enough companionship, and you may want to think about this aspect of provision for your children.

■Playthings

Buy for durability. Durable toys made of good, solid materials are expensive, but even if you have only one or two children, toys can be passed to friends, sold through small ads or saved for grandchildren! Well-made stuffed animals and wooden toys will last nearly for ever.

1. Look for toys made of natural materials: cloth, paper, leather, natural fleece, wood and metal.

2. Let children play with real things: put together a child-sized collection of pots and pans and dishes, instead of a tiny plastic kitchen.

3. Second-hand toys can be cleaned and mended. Let your child choose a new paint colour.

4. Invest in beautiful, adaptable toys like the wooden train sets made by the Swedish firm Brio. For splendid, mostly maple toys – from basic blocks to climbing frames and a wooden ironing board and iron – write to Community Playthings for their mail order catalogue.

5. Toy libraries will give your children variety and save you money. Swapping toys with friends is another idea.

6. Make playthings. Penelope Leach's *Baby and Child* (Penguin, 1979) lists good ideas, many made from 'recycled' household items.

7. Have a special box or drawer for any sort of miniature that comes your way: tiny boxes, Marmite jars, desk supplies. These always come in handy.

8. Make a dolls' house, perhaps in an old sideboard with its doors removed. Use scraps of gift wrapping paper for the walls, leftover bits of carpet for the floors. You can make – or help your child to make – much of the furniture. Toothpaste caps make lampshades, or drinking glasses for larger dolls, and all sorts of odds and ends can be put to good use.

9. A dress-up box is essential: children love long, sparkly, over-the-top clothes, so if you don't have that sort of thing to pass on pick up some at a jumble sale. They also adore funny shoes and hats. Old leather shoes can be washed in a basin of

soapy water (dry away from heat).

10. In general, stick with pencils, chalk and crayons, instead of plastic pens. And watch out for marking pens that contain chemical solvents – these can be dangerous.

11. Some children adore filling in colouring books, but they don't encourage a child's imagination like plain paper. Let children use the back of printed sheets of paper to draw on (you can save this from junk mail) or buy drawing pads made of recycled paper. Blackboards and writing slates are fun too (and good for messages).

12. All those post-paid return envelopes which come with bills can be used to play office (if you, sensibly, pay by bank giro), along with spare order forms and other bits of paper you would otherwise throw away.

13. Magazines and colour catalogues can be cut up and pasted in various ways. (Establish a specific place for used magazines or you'll find your latest *Computer World* being hacked to bits.)

14. A button box handy for sewing and mending, can be a treasure trove. So can a collection of seashells or whatever your particular passion is.

15. Build a Wendy house. This is an excellent way to use scrap wood, mouldings, carpet and wallpaper left from a bigger project.

16. Toys shouldn't be substitutes for hands–on assistance from parents. Often a child just needs a little adult aid to turn a cardboard box into a spaceship or a sturdy fruit crate into a cooker.

17. Let children join in your tasks whenever you can. They may not be able to make the same economic contribution to the

family that children did a century ago, but it's good for them to feel that they can help. They can also acquire useful skills early in life (sewing on buttons may seem great fun to an eight year old).

CHILDREN FIRST

Saving the earth is not an abstract hope. It depends on concrete acts which flow from an understanding that the natural world is precious and that we are part of it. Saving the earth also depends on an awareness of our interconnectedness, as neighbours and citizens, as parents and as the friends and neighbours of parents and their children. An increasing number of commentators believe that the welfare of children should shape social policies because children are more vulnerable to the physical and cultural environment they live in than adults are, and because their experiences as children will determine the adults they become. They are the society of the future.

One of the goals of green thinking is to show that problems are never isolated and separate, and neither are solutions. If we solve any single problem at its root, we are likely to solve other problems too. For example, if adult work were spread more evenly throughout the country, there would be more familiar adults in residential neighbourhoods during the day and children would be safer. Fewer cars and traffic calming techniques would allow children to play outdoors more. At the same time, working at or near home would dramatically reduce energy consumption.

As a mother, I often think of a maxim which comes from Native American traditions: 'We do not inherit the earth from our parents, we borrow it from our children.'

17

PETS

What role should animals play in our lives? Most children are thrilled by almost any kind of animal, and there is evidence that animals play an important role in children's emotional development. More than half the households in Britain have at least one cat or dog, and the more children in a family, the more pets we are likely to have. But city children – and often country children too – seldom have any contact with wild animals or even with the domesticated animals that provide us with food and clothing.

The dilemma is that our pets consume vast amounts of food while people starve in other parts of the world and go hungry in many parts of Britain. More than £50 million is spent simply advertising pet foods and the range of products designed to tempt our fussy furry companions is growing all the time. This is a phenomenon seen only in North America and Britain; throughout the rest of the world, cats and dogs live on scraps and leftovers, or are treated as wild animals and expected to fend for themselves.

Cats and dogs are carnivorous, and other animals have to be raised and slaughtered in order to feed them. The giant Blue Bass was hunted to near extinction in order to feed dogs and cats. Since it takes approximately 10 lb of vegetable or grain protein to produce 1 lb of animal protein, and the grain used to feed live-stock is often imported from third world countries, keeping a pet needs some serious thought.

Eighty per cent of owners buy tinned petfood, an estimated 2 billion cans every year, and packaging is another environmental cost of keeping pets. Plastic and foil pouches are even worse than tins as they cannot be recycled.

In addition, domestic pets can have a devastating impact on local wildlife. A recent report gave the results of a study of domestic cats as predators in towns and suburbs, finding that small mammals are the major prey of cats, with birds in second place, presumably because they are more difficult to catch. None the less, one-third to half of all sparrow deaths in the areas sur-veyed had been caused by house cats. This is a subject that hasn't received much attention yet, but one you should keep in mind.

CHOOSING TO KEEP A PET

Pets can fulfil a social need by offering companionship to people who live on their own and who do not have a supportive family or community network. A dog offers protection without turning your home into a fortress, not an inconsequential point for women or elderly people who live alone. What about all the little old ladies whose dog or canary is their only companion?

Is it fair to keep a large dog confined in a city flat? An unhappy, barking dog is a nuisance to neighbours and a potential danger. Britain is fortunate in not having to worry about rabies in the estimated 400,000 dog bites that occur each year, but there are any number of horrifying news reports of children mauled and permanently disfigured by previously docile animals. In spite of the British reputation as animal lovers, some 350,000 dogs are put down every year (that is nearly 1000 every day) and the RSPCA estimates that there are 500,000 unwanted dogs roaming our streets. Consider giving a home to a mongrel from a dogs' home, rather than to a highly-bred pedigree.

If you already have a cat or dog, your choice is made, and you can skip to the sections on feeding and pet care. If you are thinking about acquiring a pet, ask yourself the following questions.

▶ How will you feed your pet? Look through the section on feeding.

▶ If you want a dog, have you considered how you will deal with its excrement? Don't imagine that public paths and parks are suitable toilet facilities.

▶ What size dog will you choose? Large dogs are comparable to large cars, both in terms of expense and environmental impact.

▶ Think carefully before acquiring more than one animal. Most cats are solitary creatures and a dog will be happy with your companionship.

▶ Why do you want a pet? Security and companionship can be achieved by other means. And there are alternatives to keeping a cat or dog.

▶ Is it fair to keep a pet in a city or town, particularly if it will have to spend most of its time indoors?

▶ How do your neighbours feel about pets? Would your pet bother them?

▶ If you want a pet for the children's sake, think realistically about whether they will be able to cope with its care. Regular contact with animals on a city farm, for example, may provide a sensible, conflict-free alternative.

▶ What will you do to prevent your animal from breeding? Puppies and kittens may be sweet, but the numbers of neglected animals that have to be killed every year should give pause to any pet owner. Neutering is essential for responsible pet keeping.

▶ Can you ensure that your pet does not adversely affect local wildlife? Dogs should not be allowed to roam freely.

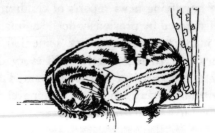

PET-KEEPING SIMPLIFIED

- Choose short-haired animals or animals with no hair.
- Keep them either indoors or out, not both.
- Don't allow them to be fussy about food.
- Keep equipment to a minimum.
- Don't allow them to procreate.

FEEDING DOGS AND CATS

As with humans, ecological eating is healthy eating. The first principle is to avoid commercial pet foods. This may come as a shock, but those packets and tins are not only expensive and wasteful, but bad for your pet. The food inside can be contaminated with lead from the soldering, and more important is heavily laced with chemical additives, flavourings, salt and even sugar, just like processed human food.

Dry commercial food is more sympathetically packaged, in cardboard or paper, and it can sometimes be bought in bulk. It is also lighter, which means lower transport costs (and energy consumption). However, it is still a highly processed food, made from the by-products of intensive meat rearing. You may find that your pets seem to be addicted to their current brand of food. American vets suggest that '. . . excessive – and costly – eating may be caused also by addiction to the chemical appetite stimulants and preservatives in fake foods'.

Semi-moist food is highest in preservatives and sugar, and the (humanly) attractive gravy which you mix with some expensive dry dog foods is actually undesirable for a dog, which should have water after a meal.

The wild ancestors of today's cats and dogs ate a very different diet from the one we expect our pets to thrive on. In the wild, cats and dogs would eat the organ meat of their prey first. It would, obviously, be raw. The closer you can replicate this diet, the healthier your pet will be. Most important, what they ate was fresh and raw – not cooked or dried and preserved with chemicals.

The scraps butchers sell for pets are often fat and gristle, not the best thing for your pet. Discuss your pet's requirements with your butcher – concentrating on liver, kidney, heart and so on. Do not aim for 'lean' meat. Cats need a fairly high intake of saturated fat. Variety is important for a balanced diet, and the butcher may be able to set aside appropriate pieces for you, or do a special deal if you buy a large amount for the freezer. Make friends with your fishmonger too.

This diet will be cheaper than your pet's present one, as well as healthier. You're not expected to buy steak for your dog! One pet writer reported that animals on a natural diet eat approximately one third less and, incidentally, produce far less waste (faeces). This is because the food is more nutritious and better digested.

The most difficult thing for most of us is that fresh and unprocessed food cannot be stored on a shelf indefinitely like a tin, and needs to be cut up (but not too much – animals are quite capable of chewing fairly large chunks of meat). If you are squeamish, perhaps you'll want to consider a vegetarian diet for your pet.

Which? reports on pet food confirm what we all know, that cats are finicky. Here are some observations on converting cats from a processed to wholefood diet. Like many cats ours were devoted to a leading brand of tinned cat food, which we supplemented with dry food. Our first switch was to a premium brand of tinned food, simply because it was nice to dish out something that was recognizably what the label claimed. We also started offering small amounts of raw meat, along with table scraps.

We gradually increased the portions of fresh offal (mainly heart, but sometimes kidneys or liver) and reduced the processed food they got. There were some failures, when they refused to touch something and howled when we refused to give them anything else, but after some months they tucked into their raw food diet with an enthusiasm that would do credit to a television commercial.

Hunger does seem to be the best sauce when trying to get cats to switch to something different. This is difficult if you are soft-hearted, when those imploring looks and plaintive meows start coming thick and fast!

One-quarter of a cat's diet can be made up of cooked cereals (brown rice for example) and grated carrot. This sounds fine to me, but I don't know how to convince the cats. Many cats, however, enjoy table scraps – everything from tossed salad to boiled potatoes. Mixing the grated vegetable into something they like works with dogs. Cats are remarkably skilful at picking out what they want and leaving the rest.

Meat can come from the supermarket during your weekly shop or buy a small amount from your butcher every couple of days. Bulk purchases can be frozen and a small amount thawed each day (it should be near room temperature when offered to your pet). One great advantage of a butcher is that you can ask for the meat to be cut into pieces for you – for freezing it could be packed in old yoghurt cartons. Some pet shops sell large bags of chopped tripe and other fresh meat for dogs.

Keep a couple of tins or a box of dried food in the cupboard for emergencies. Wholefood shops sell a few additive-free, natural products which you could try.

VEGETARIAN PETS

If you start from birth it is possible to raise a dog as a vegetarian. Although this is against canine nature, in today's world it seems a reasonable compromise, and the Vegetarian Society will provide detailed information sheets about a suitable vegetarian diet for dogs.

They do not, however, recommend a vegetarian diet for cats. A vegetarian diet is deficient in arachidonic acid, an essential fatty acid found in the structural fats of meat and fish. Because of this, the Vegetarian Society 'urges vegetarian cat owners to consider whether their beliefs are consistent with risking jeopardizing the health of any animal, or whether they should ask any animal to adapt its natural diet to suit the philosophy of the owner, no matter how noble the cause'.

In fact, a dog's diet should be only one-third meat (a good proportion of that offal), while a cat needs some three-quarters meat. The balance can be made up of grains, vegetables and the occasional egg. While even cats do not need milk (or saucers of cream), and it can be positively bad for them, small amounts of raw milk or yoghurt are desirable additions to the diet.

GROUND RULES FOR DOGS

While dogs provide companionship for the lonely and excitement for children, they are also a major social menace. The main problem is the appalling state of the country's pavements and parks. Dog faeces are not just unpleasant but dangerous too. According to the Hospital for Tropical Diseases in London up to 100 children in Britain suffer eye damage every year as a result of *Toxocara canis*, a roundworm which is transmitted in dog faeces.

About 1 million gallons of urine and 100 tons of faeces are left on our streets every day. Owners who allow their pets to foul public paths and parks are far more anti-social than young graffiti artists. Councils are moving towards more stringent controls and many parks and beaches now have dog-free areas. But the elimination of the dog licence means that controlling dogs is even more difficult than it used to be. The RSPCA is campaigning for dog registration.

Toxocara can be carried on shoes and pram wheels, and survives for several days on the floor. You might think about switching to slippers and leaving shoes at the door (a good way to avoid carrying street dirt inside, in any case). Park bikes and prams just inside the door if possible or even under shelter outside. If you have a crawling child, you'll need to take special care.

If you move house, find out whether dogs have had access to the garden. In one tragic case a little girl went blind after her family moved into a house which had been an RSPCA shelter.

AVOIDING DOG PROBLEMS

- Train your dog to defecate in a box or tray, inside the house or in your garden. Droppings could be flushed down the toilet. Dogs can also be trained to go on newspaper.
- Careful worming is important to eliminate toxocara – get advice from your vet. Faeces should be burned for two days after worming.
- Toxocara can survive in soil for over two years so you should ensure that your pet does not use the lawn as a loo, especially if you have children. Never eat while playing with a dog and take care to wash your hands afterwards.
- A pooper-scooper (pet shops stock these) is the answer while training your dog.
- A dog needs a considerable amount of exercise to stay healthy and happy. If you cannot provide this, either give the dog away or find someone else to take it out.
- See that your pet does not annoy neighbours with constant, irritable and irritating barking. If it does, you have a responsibility either to solve the problem or get rid of the dog.
- Use a lead, and do not allow your dog to approach any strangers, no matter how small and friendly the dog is. You should be even more careful if your beloved is a mastiff and particularly around children. (If someone wants to say hello to your pet they will approach you.)
- See that your pet wears a collar and tag with your name and address.

If you are a dog owner and all this seems overly severe, consider other people's small children: similar rules seem perfectly reasonable when applied to them.

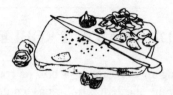

DEALING WITH FLEAS AND OTHER PESTS

Fleas can be controlled without the dangerous insecticides in commercial flea sprays, powders and collars. The first step in non-toxic flea treatment is to vacuum thoroughly: carpets, rugs, upholstery, cushions, mattresses, everything. Seal the vacuum bag in an old plastic bag and throw it away or burn it. If the problem is acute, put your bedding, pet's bedding and rugs through a hot wash. Go through this routine again after three or four days.

Next, add nutritional yeast to your pet's diet. This will make the animal taste nasty to fleas and improve its coat. Garlic will work the same trick (one mashed clove a day) and adding cider vinegar to pets' drinking water is helpful too (about a teaspoon per quart of water).

You can also make a spray by boiling up citrus peels, or mix the essential oil of lemon or orange with water to make a spray for carpets and bedding. The oil can be rubbed on to a cloth or leather collar, or you can rub a little oil into your pet's fur.

Herbal treatments can be useful, too. Pennyroyal mint is a flea-bane. Use the dried leaves to pack a fabric flea collar. You can also buy pennyroyal oil to dab on a collar or bedding; this has caused rare cases of miscarriage so be careful if you have a pregnant pet. You can also give your pet a rinse with strong (cool) pennyroyal tea after a bath.

Pets on a fresh, raw diet generally do not suffer from intestinal parasites. A daily dose of garlic is beneficial and some breeders report using nothing but garlic to prevent roundworm.

Smaller Pets

Choosing a small pet has many practical and environmental advantages. Hamsters and guinea pigs are bred in captivity, they can live happily on scraps from the kitchen, and their overall impact is slight in comparison with that of cats and dogs.

With all pets, try to cut down on the amount of commercial, packaged food you use, as well as on litter and bedding. There are books about every possible kind of pet that will have suggestions for an unprocessed diet. If you keep rodents, it's important to ensure that they do not escape into the wild, where they can throw the balance of the local ecosystem.

Although Britain signed the Convention on International Trade in Endangered Species of Wild Fauna and Flora (CITES) in 1976, many animals popular in the pet trade – from lizards, pythons and iguanas to parrots and marine fish – are rare or endangered. These animals are wild-caught and a huge proportion die during shipment. Environmentalists want a ban on the general trade in wildlife. One wildlife officer commented, 'We do not believe wild animals should be used as consumer durables.'

It may seem amusing to keep an iguana in your apartment, but by purchasing such an animal you will be supporting an unacceptable and inhumane trade. And rare animals just don't live as long in a cage in your living room as they would in their own environment. If you are choosing a bird, reptile, or tropical fish, ensure that it has been bred in captivity.

Animals In Our Lives

Wildlife groups have done a tremendous job of increasing public awareness of the importance of animal habitats and many wildlife areas have been preserved over the past few years. Everyone knows that we need green spaces in our cities. But having other living creatures around – birds, rabbits, deer, hedgehogs, fox, goats, beetles, butterflies and earwigs – is just as important as open grass for sport, trees to doze under and flowers to smell.

The ecological system of home and garden will be richer and

more successful if you have a variety of creatures in it. Sparrows and blue tits will eat insects which would otherwise be nibbling on your primroses. Frogs and toads will grow fat eating your slugs. Hens will eat kitchen scraps and produce wonderful manure for the garden.

If you feel that it is essential to share your life with some small living creature, look for alternatives. Your neighbours probably would not welcome a cockerel, but if you have a large garden there's no reason why you can't keep hens or rabbits. While city by-laws do not prohibit goats, they need a bit of room. But think about what you are going to do with hens (once they stop laying) and any baby bunnies (an unavoidable predicament). Can you face slaughtering them? Or can you sell them? How will you tell the children?

Domestic animals – goats, ducks, geese – could be raised on common land within communities. There are city farms all over Britain now, providing children and older people with a chance to experience something of the life of a farm. They also give people a chance to buy locally reared food.

Humans need contact with other creatures for emotional well-being and we need a proper picture of the ecological balances which enable us to survive on the earth. Even in the countryside the sight of a pig rolling in the dirt or a flock of chickens scratching for insects has become a rarity: intensive animal rearing sees to that. An increase in natural habitat for native animals and the keeping of domestic animals on city farms (as well as by individuals) can help to make the city a living ecosystem instead of a concrete jungle.

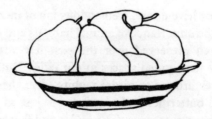

POSTSCRIPT: THE BIG PICTURE

Where do we go from here? How do we change the world around us, influence our friends, politicians and the companies that make the products we use every day? *The Green Home* is about making small changes in the way we live, but I hope you will feel inspired to get involved with some of the larger issues too.

Knowing that we *can* make a difference makes it easier to face the latest news about global warming, food safety, pesticides, hazardous waste, sustainable development, over-population, endangered species, ozone depletion and other environmental issues we hear about regularly. By understanding the connections between your own life and some of these issues, it becomes easier to care, because you feel a sense of direct involvement and impact.

You don't have to be an environmental activist in order to make a difference. The questions we need to keep in mind are simple. What do we value? What do we care about? The Worldwatch Institute puts it this way: 'In the end, individual values are what drive social change. Progress toward sustainability thus hinges on a collective deepening of our sense of responsibility to the earth and to future generations. Without a reevaluation of our personal aspirations and motivations, we will never achieve an environmentally sound global community.'

Environmental issues are given prominent coverage in newspapers and on television; there are many excellent books based on a growing body of research and campaigning groups can send you information about everything from wood treatment chemicals to aluminium in drinking water. Subscribe to one or two of the magazines listed in the Sources to keep up to date on the environmental, health and social issues that concern you. The best source of general information on environmental and social issues is the Worldwatch Institute's annual *State of the World* report, published by Earthscan.

There are often contradictory stories about an issue, so you need to be alert to what you read or hear. Assess the motives of the person or organization presenting you with information or soliciting your support. Ask where the information comes from and who paid for the research.

Writing letters to your legislative representatives, and to manufacturers and retailers is important in creating essential changes in government and business. Tell them that you care about the issues, that you are willing and eager to live a little differently in order to make change possible, and that they must do their part. Here are a few tips on communication.

▶ Give your letter a subject heading and keep it short and specific.

▶ If you have more than one complaint or subject, write separate letters so they can be directed to the right departments.

▶ Consider writing letters with several friends – you'll save time and postage.

▶ Type it if possible or at least ensure that it is legibly handwritten. Use a good quality recycled paper.

▶ A word processor makes it easy to produce letters, but personalize each one with a handwritten postscript beneath your signature and address the envelopes by hand.

▶ Make it clear that you are a voter/taxpayer/customer, so the person you have written to will want to keep you on their side.

▶ Conclude your letter with a question so the addressee will be obliged to reply.

▶ Keep a copy of everything you write.

Even better than writing letters is joining with other people in a cause you care about. You may be a member of one or more of the national pressure groups, such as the Friends of the Earth or Greenpeace, but don't forget that smaller community groups need your financial and practical support, too.

You won't find soulmates at every meeting, but you will almost certainly hit upon a group and a campaign that fits your personal interests and concerns. Developing the confidence to explain, gracefully and politely, how you feel about particular issues becomes easier when you are part of a supportive community or group.

If the idea of activism makes you nervous, don't underestimate the power of your personal example. Seeing you use terry nappies, save tea leaves for your compost heap or ride a bike to the company picnic will inevitably influence the people around you. This isn't a matter of making people feel guilty, but of showing what is possible by putting ecological principles into action.

Equally important is the example you set for your children and their friends. Take time to explain to them why you carry a string bag to the shops, and how turning off lights and putting a special blanket around the hot water tank will help to keep the earth from warming up. The other day my son asked why there were so many people in cars and where were they all going. The Department of Transport should be asking the same questions.

Summarizing the 'most important things to do' isn't easy, but here is a modest list of principles. They will not save the earth, but they will help you to live more lightly on it.

▶ Buy less and buy thoughtfully.

▶ Value the things you hold and handle and own.

▶ Pay attention to waste and gradually reduce waste in your life.

▶ Reuse and recycle whenever you can.

▶ Walk more – slow down and enjoy the world.

▶ Drive less.

▶ Have your bicycle greased and tuned, and get on it.

▶ Reduce the plastic in your life.

▶ Choose organically grown products and cut back on processed foods.

▶ Eat less meat and more grains, vegetables and fruits.

▶ Switch to non-toxic household products.

The problems discussed in *The Green Home* are complex, and realistic general solutions are not always easy to come by as they depend on cooperation between governments, business and on choices that each of us makes at home and at work. There are a remarkable number of solutions waiting in the wings for public and political acceptance. Large numbers of people will change only when it is easy to recycle, buy green cleaners and take the train rather than drive.

While green consumerism claimed that 'people's ordinary spending is the most powerful agent of change they possess' I believe that we are far more powerful as vocal parents, neighbours, co-workers and citizens. Buying is passive. We can instead choose to be active in the world, using our energy, courage and imagination to create the future we want, the future we share.

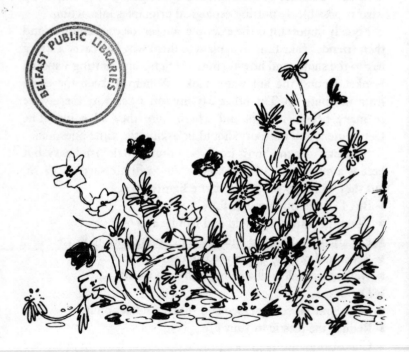

SOURCES

A resource list can never be complete – organizations come and go, new books are published and others go out of print – but this list includes campaigning groups, networks and publications I think you'll find particularly helpful. If you can recommend others, please write (care of Piatkus Books or e-mail: christensen@external.umass.edu.) and tell me about them.

RECOMMENDED ORGANIZATIONS

These groups are doing vital work in many areas relevant to *The Green Home*. Write to them for more information, join a local group and make a donation if you can.

Women's Environmental Network, Aberdeen Studios, 22 Highbury Grove, London N5 2EA, tel. 0171-354 8823. Campaigns on a range of environmental issues of particular significance to women. Produces a series of briefing papers – on issues such as chlorine, sanitary protection, packaging and pesticides – and has local groups throughout the UK. A first-rate resource for the green homemaker.

WEN also runs an information line called the Women's

Environmental Network Directory of Information, providing practical advice on the environmental impact of consumer products. Call 0171-704 6800.

Common Ground, Seven Dials Warehouse, 44 Earlham St, London WC2H 9LA, tel. 0171-379 3109. 'A small charity working to conserve nature, landscape and places with the help of people in all walks of the arts.' Contact for leaflets and information.

Friends of the Earth, 26–28 Underwood Street, London N1 7JQ, tel. 0171-490 1555. For membership enquiries ring 01582 482297. Campaigns on a wide range of issues, including recycling, pesticides, transport, rainforests and nuclear power. FoE's range of publications is considerable and includes excellent teaching packs for schools. There are FoE groups in most parts of the country; members can tell you what's going on in your area.

Greenpeace, 30–31 Islington Green, London N1 8BR, tel. 0171-354 5100. Campaigns internationally for a nuclear-free world, fresh air, clean waters, and the protection of wildlife and natural habitats.

■ Electronic Networking

An increasing amount of information on green issues is available through electronic networks and Internet newsgroups. Many environmentalists rely on fast, cheap electronic communication to stay in touch with colleagues around the world.

GreenNet, 4th Floor, 393–395 City Road, London EC1V 1NE, tel. 0171-713 1941, fax. 0171-833 1169, e-mail:support@gn.apc.org, is part of an international network which links environmental, peace and social justice groups, and interested individuals. It provides e-mail service and access to Internet.

CIX (pronounced Kicks), tel. 0181-390 8446, is a UK-based e-mail system with access to Internet.

Demon Internet Ltd, tel. 0181-371 1234, offers full direct access to Internet and e-mail.

SOURCES BY CHAPTER

■1 Time

Hochschild, Arlie, *The Second Shift* (Piatkus, 1989)

Schumacher, E. F., *Small is Beautiful: Economics as if People Mattered* (Abacus Books).

■2 What We Save And Spend

The Schumacher Circle, Foxhole, Dartington, Totnes, Devon TQ9 6EB, tel. and fax 01803 863843. This informal network of organizations, working to develop positive approaches to global environmental and social problems, includes the Schumacher Society, Intermediate Technology, the Soil Association, the New Economics Foundation and *Resurgence* magazine. Write for membership information and a publications list.

The Other Economic Summit (TOES) and the New Economics Foundation, both at First Floor, Vine Court, 112–116 Whitechapel Road, London E1 1JE, tel. 0171-377 5696. A research organization developing principles and programmes for an economics which values sustainability, good work, human well-being and self-reliance.

Advertising Standards Authority, Brook House, Torrington Place, London WC1E 7HN. This is where you write to complain about misleading or inappropriate advertising.

Thein Durning, Alan/Worldwatch Institute, *How Much is Enough?* (Earthscan, 1992). A thoughtful and thought-provoking assessment of consumerism.

LETSlink, 61 Woodcock Road, Warminster, Wilts. BA12 9DE. Write with SAE for information on Local Exchange Trading Schemes. You may find one operating in your area or if not you may want to start one.

Peter Lang, *LETS Work, Rebuilding the Local Economy* (Grover Books, 1994). Read about the principles and practice of LETS.

Ethical Investment Research Service (EIRIS), 504 Bondway Business Centre, 71 Bondway, London SW8 1SQ, tel. 0171-735 1351.

Ethical Investment Agency, FREEPOST, 9 Bramwith Road, Sheffield, S11 7EZ, tel. 0114 230 3115.

The Ecology Building Society, 18 Station Road, Crosshills, Keighley, West Yorkshire BD20 8TB, tel. 01535 635933, lends on small-scale businesses with an ecological bias, organic smallholdings and farms, and properties which will contribute to the regeneration of rural areas and inner cities. Invest in a green future.

■3 Buying with The Earth In Mind

George, Susan and Paige, Nigel, *Food for Beginners* (Airlift).

Ethical Consumer magazine, ECRA Publishing, FREEPOST MR9429, Manchester M1 8DR. This magazine is organized much like *Which?*, with a focus on ethical issues; a regular section is called Boycott News, listing new and ongoing boycotts.

Which?, Consumers' Association, 2 Marylebone Road, London NW1 4DX, tel. 0171-486 5544. The CA's advert-free publications frequently cover green consumer issues.

New Consumer, 52 Elswick Road, Newcastle upon Tyne NE4 6JH. A public interest organization focused on corporate social responsibility and consumer product analysis.

New Internationalist magazine, 120–126 Lavender Avenue, Mitcham, Surrey CR4 3HP, tel. 0181-685 0372. Covers many topics mentioned in *The Green Home* – a good source of information about ethical issues.

Pirsig, Robert, *Zen and the Art of Motorcycle Maintenance* (Vintage, 1991).

Traidcraft plc, Kingsway, Gateshead, Tyne & Wear NE11 0NE. Sells fair trade goods by mail order. Free catalogue.

Steve and Susan Hammett Recycled Stationery, Gate Farm, Fen End, Kenilworth, Warwickshire CV8 1NW, telephone and fax: 01676 533832. A noteworthy source of personal and business stationery, design and printing, and innovative paper products. Free catalogue. Send 3 first class stamps for paper samples.

Elkington, John and Hailes, Julia, *The Green Consumer Guide* (Gollancz, 1988) and *The Green Supermarket Shopping Guide* (Gollancz, 1990). *The Green Consumer Guide* has had tremendous influence on the business community as well as on public consciousness of green issues.

Wells, Phil, *The Global Consumer*, (Gollancz, 1991).

Conservatree, 36B Church Street, Caversham, Reading, Berks RG4 8AU, tel. 01734 479120. A wide range of personal and business stationery.

Paperback Limited, Unit 2, Bow Triangle Business Centre, Eleanor Street, London E3 4NP, tel. 0181-980 5580. Wholesaler and mail order supplier of business and personal stationery products and office supplies, and publishes an excellent newsletter for customers.

Animal Free Shopper, available from the Vegan Society, 7 Battle Road, St Leonard's-on-Sea, East Sussex TN37 7AA, tel. 01424 427393.

Animal Aid, The Old Chapel, Bradford Street, Tonbridge, Kent TN9 1AW, tel. 01732 364546, campaigns against factory farming and vivisection, and promotes a 'cruelty-free' lifestyle. Send large SAE for catalogue.

■4 The Three Rs: Reduce, Reuse, Recycle

Mailing Preference Service, FREEPOST 22, London W1E 7EZ. Write to have your name removed from bulk mailing lists.

Women's Environmental Network, Aberdeen Studios, 22 Highbury Grove, London N5 2EA, tel. 0171-354 8823. Support WEN's packaging 'Wrap It Up' campaign and order some 'Send It Back' labels to return unnecessary packaging to manufacturers and retailers.

Centre for Environmental Initiatives, The Old School House, Mill Lane, Carshalton, near Sutton, Surrey SM5 2JY, tel. 0181-770 6611. The group that helped make Sutton the 'green' borough.

The Original Wormery and the 'Rotol' Compost Converter, Original Organics, 49 High Street, Halberton, Tiverton, Devon EX16 7AG, tel. 0884 821432.

Save Waste & Prosper (SWAP), PO Box 19, 6–8 Great George Street, Leeds LS1 6TF, tel. 0113 2438777. Offers consultancy on recycling, energy saving and waste reduction.

McHarry, Jan, *Reuse, Repair, Recycle* (Gaia Books, 1993).

Costello, Alison, Vallely, Bernadette and Young, Josa, *The Sanitary Protection Scandal* (WEN, London, 1989).

■5 Food To Sustain Us

'Look Again at the Label' leaflet, lists of farms selling organic food and other publications from the Soil Association, 86 Colston Street, Bristol BS1 5BB, tel. 0117 9290661.

The Food Magazine and other publications from the Food Commission, Third Floor, 5–11 Worship Street, London EC2A 2BH, tel. 0171-628 7774.

The Vegetarian Society of the UK, Parkdale, Dunham Road, Altrincham, Cheshire WA14 4QG, tel. 0161 928 0793.

The Vegan Society, 7 Battle Road, St Leonard's-on-Sea, East Sussex TN37 7AA, tel. 01424 427393.

BBC Vegetarian Good Food magazine, on newstands or from PO Box 425, Woking GU21 1GP, 01483 727762.

Marshall, Janette, *Fast Food for Vegetarians* (Penguin, 1989).

Compassion in World Farming, Charles House, 5A Charles Street, Petersfield, Hants GU32 3EH, tel. 01730 264208.

The Real Meat Company Ltd, East Hill Farm, Heytesbury, Warminster, Wilts BA12 0HR, tel. 01985 840436.

Sustainable Agriculture Food and Environment Alliance (SAFE), a network of some 30 food producers and environmental organizations. 38 Ebury Street, London SW1W 0LU, tel. 0171–823 5660.

Green, Henrietta, *Henrietta Green's New Country Kitchen: The Best Produce, the Best Recipes* (Conran Octopus, 1994). British food at its best.

National Federation of City Farms, 93 Whitby Road, Brislington, Bristol BS4 3QF, tel. 0117 9719109. City farms often have goats' milk, eggs, honey and even meat for sale.

Ausubel, Kenny, *Seeds of Change* (HarperCollins, 1994).

Mabey, Richard, *Food for Free* (Collins, 1972) and *Plants with a Purpose* (Collins, 1977).

■6 Where We Live – Land And Shelter

Rackham, Oliver, *The History of the Countryside* (J. M. Dent, 1986).

Common Ground, 41 Shelton Street, London WC2H 9HJ, tel. 0171-379 3109. Charity working to conserve nature, landscape and place with the help of people in all walks of the arts.

Friends of the Earth, 26–28 Underwood Street, London N1 7JQ, tel. 0171-490 1555, produce a number of briefing papers on timber, which are aimed at professionals such as architects.

Mumford, Lewis, *The City in History* (Penguin, 1991).

Jacobs, Jane, *Cities and the Wealth of Nations* (Random House, U.S., 1985).

National Conservancy Council, Northminster House, Peterborough PE1 1UA. Advises on wildlife protection and local conservation issues.

King, Angela and Clifford, Sue, *Holding Your Ground – an action guide to local conservation* (Wildwood House, 1987).

Brookes, John, *Planting the Country Way: An Ecological Approach* (BBC Books, 1994).

'Your Council and the Environment' leaflet, a model charter covering 21 key areas including air pollution, dog nuisance, litter and rubbish collection. Available at libraries, Citizens' Advice Bureaux or by post from Angela Talboys, Room A127, Department of the Environment, Romney House, 43 Marsham Street, London SW1P 3PY, tel. 0171-276 8393.

Ecology Building Society, 18 Station Road, Cross Hills, Near Keighley, West Yorkshire BD20 7EH, tel. 01535 635933.

London Hazards Centre, Interchange Studios, Dalby Street, London NW5 3NQ, tel. 0171-267 3387.

Ecological Design Association (EDA), The British School, Slad Road, Stroud, Glos GL5 1QW, tel. 01453 765575, fax 01453 759211. A professional organization that publishes *EcoDesign* magazine and offers referrals to ecological architects and designers, as well as workshops and lectures.

Vale, Robert and Brenda, *Green Architecture* (Thames and Hudson, 1991). This book emphasizes the tremendous savings possible through energy-efficient design.

Pearson, David, *The Natural House Book* (Gaia, 1989) and *Earth to Spirit* (Gaia, 1994).

Innes, Jocasta, *The Thrifty Decorator* (Conran Octopus, 1993) includes advice on making your own paints.

Auro Organic Paint Supplies Ltd, Unit 1, Goldstones Farm, Ashdon, Saffron Walden, Essex CB10 2ET, tel. 01799 584 888.

Harland, Edward, *Eco-Renovation* (Resurgence Books, 1994). This useful book is written by a British architect. Order through your bookshop or from the Schumacher Book Service.

The Building Bookshop, 26 Store Street, London WC1E 7BT, tel. 0171-637 3151. Reference material and manufactures' literature.

The Healthy House, Cold Harbour, Ruscombe, Stroud, Glos GL6 6DA, tel. 01453 752216, fax 01453 753533. This mail order catalogue specializes in products for people suffering from allergies and environmental illness. The range includes non-toxic paints, water filters and computer accessories.

■7 Energy Choices

Centre for Alternative Technology, Llwyngwern Quarry, Machynlleth, Powys SY20 9AZ, tel. 01654 702400. Send £1 and a large SAE for their extensive mail order booklist. Exhibitions and displays open to visitors; weekend courses.

Neighbourhood Energy Action, St Andrew's House, 90–92 Pilgrim Street, Newcastle upon Tyne NE1 6SG, tel. 0191 261 5677. Promotes energy efficiency to combat fuel poverty.

Bristol Energy Centre and the Centre for Sustainable Energy, The Create Centre, B-bond Warehouse, Smeaton Road, Bristol BS1 6XN, tel. 0117 9304097. Concentrates on energy saving and fuel poverty, with draught-proofing team.

Practical Alternatives is a business run by David Huw Stephens, Tir Gaia Solar Village, Rhayader, Powys LD6 5DX, tel. 01597 810929, which markets practical and durable goods to help people conserve the earth's resources. Practical Alternatives is also building a solar village. Send SAE for details.

Domestic Paraphernalia Co., Unit 15, Marine Business Centre, Dock Road, Lytham, Lancs FY8 5JA, tel. 01253 736334, for clothes airer/dryer.

Intermediate Technology Development Group, 103–105 Southampton Row, London WC1B 4HH, tel. 0171-436 9761.

Choosing and Using a New Gas Cooker or Central Heating Boiler, Gas Consumers Council, Abford House, 15 Wilton Road, London SW1V 1LT, tel. 0171-931 0977.

Green computer peripherals: Nighthawk Electronic Ltd, FREEPOST, Saffron Walden, Essex CB11 3BR, tel. 01799 540881, fax 01799 541713.

Vale, Robert and Brenda, *Green Architecture* (Thames and Hudson, 1991). Practising architects, the Vales have written a number of books on environmentally sound buildings. Their home in Nottinghamshire is self-sufficient in water, waste treatment, heating and electricity.

■8 Out And About: How We Get Around

Sustrans (Paths for People), 35 King Street, Bristol BS1 4DZ, tel. 0117 9268893, fax 0117 9294173. Campaigns for sustainable transport in Britain, developing a network of cycling and walking paths throughout the country, and promoting the idea of safe, flexible, environmentally sound transport. Join the campaign and get a map of paths in use and in progress.

Transport 2000, 10 Melton Street, London NW1 2EJ, tel. 0171-388 8386. Campaigns for efficient and comprehensive public transportation.

Ballantine, Richard, *Richard's New Bicycle Book* (Pan, 1990).

RSPA Bicycle Owner's Handbook, available from the Royal Society for the Prevention of Accidents, Cannon House, The Priory, Queensway, Birmingham B4 6BS, tel. 0121 200 2461, is a useful guide.

Ramblers' Association, 1/5 Wandsworth Road, London SW8 2XX, tel. 0171-582 6878. A membership organization supporting ramblers' rights, and organizing events and walking holidays.

Centre for the Advancement of Responsive Travel (CART), 70 Dry Hill Park Road, Tonbridge, Kent TN10 3BX. Aims at creating better cross-cultural understanding through workshops for those planning long-distance trips.

Tourism Concern, Southlands College, Roehampton Institute, Wimbledon Parkside, London SW19 5NN, tel. 0181-944 0464. Promotes the understanding of the impact of tourism on the environment and on people living in holiday areas.

The Outward Bound Trust, Chestnut Field, Regent Place, Rugby CV21 2PJ, tel. 01788 560423.

Earthwatch, Belsyre Court, 57 Woodstock Road, Oxford OX2 6HU, tel. 01865 311600.

Working Weekends on Organic Farms (WWOOF), 19 Bradford Road, Lewes, Sussex BN7 1RB, tel. 01273 476286.

Elkington, John and Hailes, Julia, *Holidays that Don't Cost the Earth* (Gollancz, 1992). A guide to green (or greenish) holidays, with an emphasis on ecotourism. Read this before you plan your next trip.

Weekend Walks in Britain (AA Publishing, 1994). A ringbinder with suggestions for 200 walks and related maps. Take the sections you need with you as you ramble.

9 The Air We Breathe

National Society For Clean Air, 136 North Street, Brighton BN1 1RG, tel. 01273 326313.

Friends of the Earth, 26–28 Underwood Street, London N1 7JQ, tel. 0171-490 1555. Send SAE for publications list which includes leaflets on the effects of ozone depletion, methyl bromide, industrial solvents and common air pollutants.

Good Air Quality in Your Home, Department of the Environment, PO Box 151, London E15 2HF, fax 0181-533 1618.

10 Water

The Centre for Alternative Technology in Powys, *see* p. 300.

National Rivers Authority has regional offices – check your telephone directory – which can answer questions, and provide you with leaflets on how to avoid chlorinated solvent and oil pollution. Call the NRA's free emergency hotline to report suspected pollution incidents: 0800 80 70 60 (do not use this number for general enquiries).

Marine Conservation Society, 9 Gloucester Road, Ross-on-Wye, Herefordshire HR9 5BU, tel. 01989 566017.

11 Health and Healing

The Environmental Health Department of your district council should be able to give advice on asbestos, lead in paint, radon, chemical safety (e.g. pesticide spraying in parks) and proper disposal of hazardous chemicals.

Bothered by Noise? What you can do about it, Department of the Environment, PO Box 151, London E15 2HF, fax 0181-533 1618.

British Allergy Foundation, St Bartholomew's Hospital, London EC1A 7BE. Send SAE for leaflets on coping with allergies in the home.

What Doctors Don't Tell, 4 Wallace Road, London N1 2PG. Monthly, advert-free newsletter which aims to tell the whole truth about modern medicine, with full discussion of alternative views. Write for current subscription details.

Bates, W. H., *Better Eyesight Without Glasses* (Grafton, 1979).

Goodrich, Janet, *Natural Vision Improvement* (David & Charles, 1987).

Pearse, Innes H. and Crocker, Lucy H., *The Peckham Experiment, a Study in The Living Structure of Society* (Scottish Academic Press, 1985) and the Pioneer Health Centre Ltd, 'Camolin,' Birtley Rise, Bramley, Guildford GU5 0HZ.

Halvolsen, Brian, *The Natural Dentist* (Century Arrow, 1986).

Woodham, Anne, *HEA Guide to Complementary Medicine and Therapies* (Health Education Authority, 1994). An excellent guide to dozens of therapies, rating them for popularity, medical credibility, scientific research and availability. It lists licensing bodies and gives advice on finding a practitioner.

Institute of Complementary Medicine, PO Box 194, London SE16 1QZ, tel. 0171-237 5165. Another source of referrals to practitioners.

Green Burial – the DIY guide to law and practice, The Natural Death Centre, 20 Heber Road, London NW2 6AA, tel. 0181-208 2853. Albery, N., Elliot, G. and Elliot, J. (eds), *The Natural Death Handbook* (Virgin, 1993). Also contact the AB Wildlife Trust, 7 Knox Road, Harrogate, North Yorkshire HG1 3EF. tel. 01423 530900.

■12 The Non-Toxic Home

London Hazards Centre, 3rd Floor, Headland House, 308 Grays Inn Road, London WC1X 8DS, tel. 0171-837 5605. Researches alternatives to various indoor environmental hazards, from VDU radiation to timber treatments.

Little Green Shop, 16 Gardner Street, Brighton, East Sussex BN1 1UP, tel. 01273 571221. Sells environmentally friendly, green, cruelty-free household products. Retail and mail order.

■ 13 Reducing Radiation

National Radiological Protection Board (NRPB), Chiltern, Didcot, Oxon OX11 0RQ, tel. 01235 831600. Provides information on UK radon surveys.

The Department of the Environment (DoE) produce a leaflet called *The Householder's Guide to Radon*. For a copy, tel. 0171-276 0900.

The Food Commission, Third Floor, 5-11 Worship Street, London EC2A 2BH, tel. 0171-628 7774. The FC's *Food Magazine* is a good source of information about recent research and the current legal position on food irradiation.

Brodeur, Paul, *The Great Power Line Coverup* (Little, Brown, New York, 1993). Articles based on the book were published in the *New Yorker* magazine, raising public consciousness of the dangers posed by electromagnetic radiation.

Webb, Tony, *Radiation and Your Health* (Camden Press, 1988). A matter-of-fact guide to radiation hazards and steps you can take to protect yourself.

■ 14 Light

True-Lite fluorescent tubes and light units are available by post from SML, Unit 1, Riverside Business Centre, Victoria Street, High Wycombe, Bucks HP11 2LT, tel. 01494 448727. Write or telephone for their information pack and price list.

■ 15 Creating A Garden

Henry Doubleday Research Association (HDRA), National Centre for Organic Gardening, Ryton-on-Dunsmore, Coventry CV8 3LG, tel. 01203 303517. Every organic gardener should join this organization. Membership includes a quarterly newsletter, free gardening advice and unlimited entry to Ryton Gardens. Send off for their publications list.

The Soil Association (Organic Food and Farming Centre), 86 Colston Street, Bristol BS1 5BB, tel. 0117 9290661. The leading UK organization for organic farming, which gives advice to consumers on obtaining organic foods from local farms, and has an extensive list of publications and books available by mail.

There are many excellent gardening books that emphasize organic techniques. The ones mentioned here offer something special for the ecological gardener.

Jeavons, John and Cox, Carol, *Lazy-Bed Gardening, the quick and dirty guide* (1993) and Jeavons, John, *How to Grow More Vegetables (than you ever thought possible on less land than you can imagine)* (Ten Speed Press, 1985 – distributed by Airlift), the classic guide to biodynamic gardening. Available from the HDRA.

Harper, Peter, *The Natural Garden Book* (Gaia, 1994).

The Friends of the Earth Guide to Peat Alternatives, *Gardening without Peat* leaflet (FoE, 1990). The use of peat is destroying Britain's wetlands; this guide will help you improve your soil with other plant materials.

Organic Gardening Magazine – order through your newsagent, or direct from PO Box 4, Wiveliscombe, Taunton, Somerset TA4 2QY, tel. 01984 623998.

Elm Farm Research Centre (Organic Advisory Service), Hamstead Marshall, Newbury, Berks RG15 0HR, tel. 01488 658298. Comprehensive soil analysis.

Suffolk Herbs, Monk Farm, Pantlings Lane, Kelvedon, Essex CO5 9PJ, tel. 01376 572456. This seed company is too good to miss, with its beautiful mail order catalogue and wide selection of seeds (herbs, unusual vegetables, wild flowers), organic products and books.

Jackman, Leslie, *The Wild Bird Garden* (Souvenir Press, 1992). A detailed, illustrated guide to making your garden appealing to birds, with information on feeding birds in winter.

Royal Society for the Protection of Birds (RSPB), The Lodge, Sandy, Bedfordshire SG19 2DL, tel. 01767 680551. The RSPB's free leaflets cover all aspects of encouraging birds, from proper feeding to providing birdhouses. Enclose SAE with your request.

The Centre for Alternative Technology in Powys, *see* p. 300.

Wildlife Trusts, The Green, Nettleham, Lincoln LN2 2NR, tel. 01522 544400. A nationwide network of local trusts working to protect wildlife in town and country. Membership includes a subscription to *Natural World*.

NPK Landlife, 40 Farlands Drive, East Didsbury, Manchester M20 5GB, tel. 0161 794 9314, fax 0161 794 8072. This charitable trust promotes the creation of natural habitats, and sells seeds and native bulbs as well as a range of publications.

Ausubel, Kenny, *Seeds of Change* (HarperCollins, 1994).

■ 16 Nurturing Our Children

Foresight, 28 The Paddock, Godalming, Surrey GU7 1XD is an organization devoted to pre-natal care. Send SAE for information on membership, courses and affiliated doctors, and read the Foresight guide, *Planning for a Healthy Baby*, by Belinda Barnes and Suzanne Bradley (Century, 1990).

Association for Improvements in the Maternity Services (AIMS). Send an SAE to 10 Topcliffe Drive, Acklam, Middlesbrough, Cleveland TS5 8HL for a free copy of *What is AIMS?* and their publication list.

National Childbirth Trust (NCT), Alexandra House, Oldham Terrace, London W3 6NH, tel. 0181-992 8637. Call or write for their publications list.

Independent Midwives Association, Nightingale Cottage, Shamblehurst Lane, Botley, Hants SO32 2BY. Lobbies for the return of the traditional role of the midwife. Send a SAE for register of independent midwives.

Odent, Michel, *Birth Reborn: What Childbirth Should Be* (Souvenir Press, 1994), *Entering the World* (Marion Boyars, 1983) and *Primal Health* (Century, 1986).

Primal Health Research Centre, 29 Roderick Road, London NW3 2NP. Michel Odent, the obstetrician who pioneered natural birth techniques in Pithviers, France, works with doctors and health professionals around the world to produce excellent studies of ecological health issues. Annual membership includes a thoughtful quarterly newsletter.

Lawrence Beech, Beverley, *Who's Having Your Baby?* (Bedford Square Press, 1991). A practical, rather brusque guide to getting the birth you want.

La Leche League of Great Britain, BM Box 3424, London WC1N 3XX, tel. 0171-242 1278. Offers advice and runs local support groups around the country. Their classic book *The Art of Breastfeeding* is available by mail order, along with a wide range of other publications: from LLB, 160 Blenheim Street, Hull HU5 3PN.

Palmer, Gabrielle, *The Politics of Breastfeeding* (Pandora, 1988). This startling book should be read by every prospective parent.

National Association of Nappy Services (NANS), St George House, Hill Street, Birmingham B5 4AN, tel. 0121 693 4949. Call to find out your nearest nappy washing service.

First Choice International, Chenley Hall, Rectory Lane, Chenley, Radlett, Herts WD7 9AN, tel. 01923 859476, produce reusable nappies. Mail order, and ask for details of retail stockists.

Liedloff, Jean, *The Continuum Concept* (Penguin, 1986) and the Liedloff Continuum Network, 10 Headley Way, Oxford OX3 0LT.

Jackson, Deborah, *Three in a Bed* (Bloomsbury, 1994).

The Food Commission, Third Floor, 5–11 Worship Street, London EC2A 2BH, tel. 0171-628 7774, publishes excellent pamphlets and books on healthy eating, including the *Nursery Food Book* by Mary Whiting and Tim Lobstein (Edward Arnold, 1992).

Chaitow, Leon, *Vaccination and Immunisation: Dangers, Delusions and Alternatives* (C. W. Daniel, 1987).

Kenton, Lesley, *Nature's Child: Guide, Nourish and Protect Your Child the Gentle Way* (Ebury Press, 1993).

Community Playthings, Darvell, Robertsbridge, East Sussex TN32 5DR, tel. 01580 880 626. Free catalogue.

Carey, Diana and Large, Judy, *Festivals, Family and Food* (Hawthorn Press, Stroud, 1982).

Leach, Penelope, *Children First* (Penguin, 1994). This excellent book argues that society, as well as individual parents, should truly put the needs of children first, and use the welfare of *all* children as a measure of our social progress.

■17 Pets

Vegetarian Society of the UK, Parkdale, Dunham Road, Altrincham, Cheshire WA14 4QG, tel. 0161 928 0793. Write with SAE for guidelines on a vegetarian diet for your dog.

Royal Society for the Prevention of Cruelty to Animals (RSPCA), Causeway, Horsham, West Sussex RH12 1HG, tel. 01403 264181 provides information on appropriate pet-keeping and sterilization options.

British Homoeopathic Association, 27a Devonshire Street, London W1N 1RJ, tel. 0171-935 2163, can refer you to a homoeopathic veterinarian.

BIBLIOGRAPHY

MAIL ORDER BOOK SUPPLIERS

Books for a Change, 52 Charing Cross Road, London WC2H OBB, tel. 0171-836 2315: email orders @ecobooks.demon.co.uk.

The Food Commission, Third Floor, 5/11 Worship Street, London EC2A 2BH, tel. 0171-628 7744.

Henry Doubleday Research Association (HDRA), Ryton on Dunsmore, Coventry CV8 3LG, tel. 01203 303517.

Schumacher Book Service, Ford House, Hartland, Bideford, Devon EX39 6EE, tel. 01237 441621.

Soil Association, 86 Colston Street, Bristol BS1 5BB, tel. 0117 9290661.

Women's Environmental Network, Aberdeen Studios, 22 Highbury Grove, London N5 2EA, tel. 0171-354 8823.

THE BOOKS

OP means, sadly, out of print. These books can often be obtained from your local library or through inter-library loan.

Alexander, Christopher et al, *A Pattern Language* (Oxford University Press, New York, 1978).

Andruss, Van et al (eds), *Home! A Bioregional Reader* (Philadelphia, PA, New Society Publishers, 1990).

Ausubel, Kenny, *Seeds of Change* (HarperCollins, 1994).

Ballantine, Richard, *Richard's New Bicycle Book* (Pan, 1990).

Barnes, Belinda and Bradley, Suzanne Gail, *Planning for a Healthy Baby* (Century, 1990).

Bates, W. H., *Better Eyesight Without Glasses* (Grafton, 1979).

Beech, Beverley Lawrence, *Who's Having Your Baby?* (Bedford Square Press, 1991).

Berry, Wendell, *The Landscape of Harmony* (Five Seasons Press, 1987).

Bertell, Rosalie, *No Immediate Danger: Prognosis for a Radioactive Earth* (Women's Press, 1985).

Brodeur, Paul, *The Zapping of America* (W. W. Norton, New York, 1977). OP

Brookes, John, *Planting the Country Way: An Ecological Approach* (BBC Books, 1994).

Bryan, Felicity, *The Town Gardener's Companion* (Penguin, 1983). OP

Button, John, *New Green Pages* (Macdonald Optima, 1990); *Green Fuse* (Quartet Books, 1990).

Campbell, Rona and Macfarlane, Alison, *Where to be born? The Debate and the Evidence* (National Perinatal Epidemiology Unit, Radcliffe Infirmary, Oxford, 1987).

Cannon, Geoffrey and Lawrence, Felicity, *Additives: Your Complete Survival Guide* (Century, 1986). OP

Canter, David, Canter, Kay and Swan, Daphne, *The Cranks Recipe Book* (Orion, 1993).

Capra, Fritjof, *The Turning Point* (Fontana, 1983).

Chaitow, Leon, *Vaccination and Immunization: Dangers, Delusions and Alternatives* (C. W. Daniel, 1987).

Chapman, Carolyn, *Style on a Shoestring, a Guide to Conspicuous Thrift* (Hutchinson, 1984). OP

Carey, Diana and Large, Judy, *Festivals, Family and Food* (Hawthorn Press, Stroud, 1982).

Costello, Alison, Vallely, Bernadette and Young, Josa, *The Sanitary Protection Scandal* (WEN, London, 1989).

Dadd, Debra Lynn, *Nontoxic, Natural and Earthwise* (J. P. Tarcher, 1990); *The Nontoxic Home and Office* (J. P. Tarcher, 1992); *Sustaining the Earth: How to Choose Products that are Environmentally Safe* (Hearst Books, 1994).

Davidson, John, *Radiation: What it is, How it Affects Us and What We Can Do About It* (C. W. Daniel, 1986); *Subtle Energy* (C. W. Daniel, 1988).

Davis, Patricia, *Aromatherapy: An A–Z* (C. W. Daniel, 1988).

Dudley, Nigel and Stickland, Sue, *G is for ecoGarden An A–Z Guide to an Organically Healthy Garden* (Gaia Books, 1991).

Elkind, David, *The Hurried Child* (Addison-Wesley, Reading, Mass., 1988).

Elkington, John and Hailes, Julia, *The Green Consumer Guide* (Gollancz, 1988) and *The Green Consumer's Supermarket Shopping Guide* (Gollancz, 1989).

Ewald, Ellen, *Recipes for a Small Planet* (Ballantine, New York, 1973). OP

Fisher, Jeffrey A., *The Plague Makers* (Simon & Schuster, 1994).

Friends of the Earth, *Don't Throw It All Away: Guide to Waste Reduction and Recycling* (FoE, 1992); *Gardening Without Peat* (FoE, 1990).

Frisch, Monica, *Directory for the Environment: Organisations, Campaigns and Initiatives in the British Isles* (Merlin Press, 1994).

Gaskin, Ina May, *Babies, Breastfeeding and Bonding* (Bergin & Garvey, New York, 1987). Available from the La Leche League.

Gear, Alan, *The New Organic Food Guide* (J. M. Dent, 1987).

Goodrich, Janet, *Natural Vision Improvement* (David & Charles, 1987). OP

Grant, Doris and Joice, Jean, *Food Combining for Health* (Thorsons, 1991).

Green, Henrietta (ed.), *British Food Finds 1987* (Rich & Green, 1987). OP; *RAC Food Routes* (George Philip & Co., 1988) OP; *Food Lovers Guide to Britain* (BBC Books, 1985); *New Country Kitchen: The Best Produce, the Best Recipes* (Conran Octopus, 1994).

Grigson, Jane, *Vegetable Book* (Michael Joseph, 1991); *Fruit Book* (Michael Joseph, 1991).

Hardyment, Christina, *From Mangle to Microwave: Mechanization of the Household* (Polity Press, 1990).

Harland, Edward, *Eco-Renovation* (Resurgence Books, 1994).

Harper, Peter et al. *The Natural Garden Book* (Gaia Books, 1994).

Illich, Ivan, *Limits to Medicine* (Marion Boyars, 1976).

Inch, Sally, *Birthrights: Parents' Guide to Modern Childbirth* (Green Print, 1989).

Innes, Jocasta, *The Pauper's Homemaking Book* (Penguin, 1976) OP and *The Thrifty Decorator* (Conran Octopus, 1993).

Jackson, Deborah, *Three in a Bed* (Bloomsbury, 1994).

Jeavons, John, *Grow More Vegetables (than you ever thought possible on less land than you can imagine)* (Ten Speed Press, Berkeley, CA, USA, 1982).

Kenton, Lesley, *Ageless Ageing: The Natural Way to Stay Young* (Century Arrow, 1986); *The Biogenic Diet* (Century, 1986) OP; *Ultrahealth* (Ebury Press, 1984) OP; *Nature's Child: Guide, Nourish and Protect Your Child the Gentle Way* (Ebury Press, 1993).

Kenton, Lesley and Kenton, Susannah, *Raw Energy* (Vermilion, 1994).

King, Angela and Clifford, Sue, *Holding Your Ground – an action guide to local conservation* (Wildwood House, 1987).

Kitto, Dick, *Planning the Organic Vegetable Garden* (Thorsons, 1986); *Composting* (Thorsons, 1988). OP

Kitzinger, Sheila, *Woman's Experience of Childbirth* (Penguin, 1987); *Freedom and Choice in Childbirth* (Penguin, 1988).

Kitzinger, Sheila and Davis, J. (eds) *Place of Birth* (Oxford University Press, 1978). OP

Kruger, Anna, *H is for ecoHome* (Gaia Books, 1991).

La Leche League, *The Art of Breastfeeding* (available from La Leche League, see Sources).

Lang, Peter, *LETS Work, Rebuilding the Local Economy* (Grover Books, 1994).

Larkcom, Joy, *Vegetables from Small Gardens* (Faber, 1976) OP; *Salads the Year Round* (Hamlyn, 1980) OP; *The Salad Garden* (F. Lincoln, 1994).

Lazarus, Pat, *Keep Your Pet Healthy the Natural Way* (Keats, 1986).

Leach, Penelope, *Baby and Child* (Penguin, 1979).

Lewith, George T., and Kenyon, Julian N. *Clinical Ecology* (Thorsons, 1985). OP

Liedloff, Jean, *The Continuum Concept* (Penguin, 1989).

Lobstein, Tim, *The Food Commission, Children's Food* (Unwin Hyman, 1988). Available from the Food Commission – see Sources.

Lobstein, Tim and Dibb, Sue, *Green Detective at the Takeaway* (Wayland, 1991).

Loewenfeld, Claire, *Herb Gardening* (Faber, 1970).

Longacre, Doris, *Living More With Less* (Lion Publishing, 1987).

Mabey, Richard, *Food for Free* (Collins, 1972), and *Plants with a Purpose* (Collins, 1977).

McHarry, Jan, *Reuse, Repair, Recycle* (Gaia Books, 1993).

Makkar, Lali and Ince, Mary, *How to Cut Your Fuel Bills* (Kogan Page, 1982). OP

Mander, Jerry, *Four Arguments for the Elimination of Television* (Morrow, New York, 1978). OP

Mendelsohn, Robert, *How to Raise a Healthy Child in Spite of Your Doctor* (Contemporary Books, Chicago, 1984).

Monro, Jean and Mansfield, Peter, *Chemical Children* (Century, 1987). OP

Montessori, Maria, *The Discovery of the Child* (Clio Press, 1988).

Moore Lappe, Frances, *Diet for a Small Planet* (Ballantine, New York, 1982). OP

Moore Lappe, Frances and Collins, Joseph, *Food First* (Souvenir Press, 1980).

Murphy, Dervla, *Race to the Finish? The Nuclear Stakes* (John Murray, 1981); *Muddling through in Madagascar* (Arrow Books, 1990); *In Ethiopia with a Mule* (Flamingo, 1994); *Where the Indus is Young* (Flamingo, 1995).

Odent, Michel, *Entering the World* (Marion Boyars, 1989); *Birth Reborn* (Souvenir Press, 1994).

Ott, John, *Light, Radiation and You* (Devin, New York, 1985); *Health and Light* (Ariel, GA, 1990).

Palmer, Gabrielle, *The Politics of Breastfeeding* (Pandora, 1988).

Patterson, Walter, *Nuclear Power* (Penguin, 1976) OP; *Going Critical* (Paladin, 1985). OP

Pearse, Innes H. and Lucy H., *The Peckham Experiment* (Allen & Unwin, 1943; Scottish Academic Press, 1985).

Pearson, David, *The Natural House Book* (Conran Octopus, 1994) and *Earth to Spirit* (Gaia, 1994).

Porritt, Jonathon, *Seeing Green* (Blackwell, 1984); *The Coming of the Greens* (Collins, 1988). OP

Rifkin, Jeremy, *Time Wars: The Primary Conflict in Human History* (Simon & Schuster, New York, 1989).

Rivers, Patrick, *Stolen Future: How to Rescue the Earth for our Children* (Green Print, 1988).

Rivers, Patrick and Shirley, *Diet for a Small Island* (Turnstone, 1981). OP

Roddick, Anita, *Body and Soul* (Ebury, 1991).

Rousseau, David, *Your Home, Your Health and Your Well-Being* (Ten Speed Press, Berkeley, Cal., 1988).

Sandwith, Hermione and Stainton, Sheila, *National Trust Manual of Housekeeping* (Penguin, 1993).

Schulman, Martha Rose, *The Vegetarian Feast* (Thorsons, 1982) OP; *Fast Vegetarian Feasts* (Thorsons, 1983).

Schumacher, E. F., *Small is Beautiful* (Vintage, 1993).

Sekers, Simone, *Fine Food* (Hodder & Stoughton, 1987) OP; *National Trust Book of Fruit and Vegetable Cookery* (National Trust, 1991).

Seymour, John, *The Forgotten Arts* (Dorling Kindersley, 1984) OP; *Changing Lifestyles: Living as though the World Mattered* (Gollancz, 1991).

Seymour, John and Girardet, Herbert, *Blueprint for a Green Planet* (Dorling Kindersley, 1988).

Smith, Drew and Mabey, David (eds), *The Good Food Directory* (Consumers' Association, 1987). OP

Smyth, Bob, *City Wildspace* (Hilary Shipman, 1987).

Solomon, Juliet, *Green Parenting* (Optima, 1990). OP

Stanway, Andrew and Penny, *Breast is Best* (Pan Books, 1983).

Thevenin, Tine, *The Family Bed* (Avery, New York, 1987). Available from La Leche League.

Thomas, Anna, *The New Vegetarian Epicure* (Penguin, 1991).

Tisserand, Robert, *The Art of Aromatherapy* (C. W. Daniel, 1977) and *Aromatherapy for Everyone* (Penguin, 1990).

Vale, Brenda and Robert, *Green Architecture* (Thames & Hudson, 1994).

Vallely, Bernadette, *1001 Ways to Save the Planet* (WEN Penguin, 1990).

Vallely, Bernadette, Aldridge, Felicity and Davis, Lorna, *Green Living* (WEN Thorsons, 1991).

Venolia, Carol, *Healing Environments* (Celestial Arts, Berkeley, CA, 1988).

Webb, Tony and Collingwood, Robin, *Radiation and Your Health* (Camden Press, 1988).

Webb, Tony and Lang, Tim, *Food Irradiation: The Facts* (Thorsons, 1987).

Worldwatch Institute, Brown Lester et al, *State of the World 1994* (Earthscan, London, 1994).

Yudkin, John, *Pure, White and Deadly* (Penguin, 1988). OP

MAGAZINES

EcoDesign from The Ecological Design Association, The British School, Slad Road, Stroud, Glos GL5 1QW, tel. 01453 765575.

The Ecologist, Subscriptions Department, Worthyvale Manor Farm, Camelford, Cornwall PL32 9TT, tel. 01840 212711. Important stuff, but heavy going for the casual reader.

Ethical Consumer, 16 Nicholas Street, Manchester M1 4EJ, tel. 0161 237 1630.

The Food Magazine, The Food Commission, Third Floor, 5–11 Worship Street, London EC2A 2BH, tel. 0171-628 7774.

The Living Earth, The Soil Association Ltd, 86–88 Colston Street, Bristol BS1 5BB, tel. 0117 9290661.

New Consumer Briefing, subscriptions from 52 Elswick Road, Newcastle upon Tyne NE4 6JH, tel. 0191 272 1148.

The New Internationalist, Subscription Offices, 120–126 Lavender Avenue, Mitcham, Surrey CR4 3HP, tel. 0181-685 0372.

Resurgence, Subscriptions Department, Salem Cottage, Trelin, Bodmin, Cornwall PL30 3HZ, tel. 01208 851304.

INDEX

ABOUT THE AUTHOR

Karen Christensen was born in 1957, the peak year of consumer satisfaction in the US. She was educated in Minnesota and Surrey, and emigrated to England after finishing university in California. She worked in publishing before writing *Home Ecology* and now, in addition to her own writing and journalism, runs a business producing academic reference books.

She has taught at University of California Santa Barbara and the City Literary Institute in London and given workshops in the UK and US. She helped found the Women's Environmental Network and the Ecological Design Association, was a UK Green Party speaker on women's issues (1990–1) and has been an adviser to the Worldwatch Institute and the People-Centered Development Forum.

Her first children's book, *Rachel's Roses*, was published by Barefoot Books in 1995 and she is working on *A Smaller Circle: the search for community* and on *Move Your Message!*, a guide to communication skills for people who want to make the world a better place.

After many years in London she now lives in a small country town – where composting is easy but public transport hard to come by – with her husband, anthropologist David Levinson, and her children, Tom and Rachel.